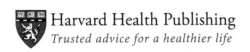

Harvard Health Publishing

Trusted advice for a healthier life

Dear Reader,

Have you ever admired a shiny, high-tech piece of exercise equipment or longed for fancy new workout gear? Even before COVID-19, Americans spent nearly $4 billion a year on home exercise equipment. In 2020, as the pandemic raged, that amount skyrocketed to $5.5 billion, a 40% increase. But here's the irony: the best piece of exercise equipment ever invented is absolutely free. It's your own body! With body-weight exercise, you don't need any equipment, because your body itself provides the weight as you move against the force of gravity.

There was a time when most of the exercise people did qualified as body-weight exercise. Many children of the 1960s will recall school gym classes that consisted largely of calisthenics like push-ups, sit-ups, and jumping jacks, which are classic body-weight exercises. But things changed in the following decades, as a proliferation of gyms brought us treadmills, Stairmasters, weight machines, and an ever-expanding array of smaller equipment, from kettlebells to Bosus. We began doing workouts tailored to a specific apparatus, like step class or Spin.

All of that came to a crashing halt with COVID-19. The pandemic shuttered gyms for months. Most people had no choice but to work out at home, and exercise equipment was nearly as scarce as toilet paper. A new set of hand weights was hard to find, used ones were selling for more than double their original price, and Peloton bikes were on back order for months. Suddenly, a lot of people rediscovered body-weight exercise.

To be fair, body-weight training was already making something of a comeback. Gyms liked the fact that body-weight exercise was economical to offer. But in 2021, it jumped to No. 3 on the American College of Sports Medicine's annual fitness trends report, right behind online training and exercise using wearable technology—all three, not coincidentally, being suitable for gym-free workouts. Body-weight exercise even outranked high-intensity interval training and yoga.

Although body-weight exercise requires no special equipment, it can provide an excellent, well-rounded workout. Because you're working against resistance, it builds strength by definition. The exercises in this report will also increase muscle power (the speed with which you can execute a move), boost cardio fitness, improve balance and coordination, rev up your metabolism, and enhance flexibility and body awareness—and you don't even have to drive to the gym or buy equipment! So, let's get started.

Elizabeth Pegg Frates, M.D.
Medical Editor

Michele Stanten
Fitness Consultant

Harvard Health Publishing | Harvard Medical School | 4 Blackfan Circle, 4th Floor | Boston, MA 02115

What is body-weight exercise?

Every time you get up from a chair or climb a flight of stairs, you're doing a simple type of body-weight exercise—a form of physical activity in which you're moving your body against the resistance of gravity. This can take the form of equipment-free cardio exercise or strength training in which you use your body itself as a weight.

Body-weight training has a long history, dating back to ancient Greece and possibly earlier. The Greeks prized physical fitness and believed a healthy mind required a healthy body. They established the Olympic games for the pursuit of sporting excellence and were known for their rigorous training methods. The original Olympic athletes practiced body-weight exercise not because they lacked objects to provide weight. (Their training regimens included bending and straightening metal bars, lifting boulders, and pulling ploughs.) Rather, they included body-weight training because it was effective. For example, they did push-ups, which require strength not only in the upper arms, but also the core, in order to hold the body straight. They also practiced running in sand—a high-resistance exercise that built leg muscles and strengthened the cardiovascular system.

In modern times, body-weight exercise has been a mainstay of training for gymnasts and soldiers. Hours of lifting, flipping, and swinging their bodies through the air—with or without equipment—make possible the stunning physiques and amazing feats of gymnasts. For the military, calisthenics are both convenient and effective. Active-duty personnel can perform body-weight exercises even in remote outposts with no special equipment. And for those stuck at home during the pandemic, body-weight exercise provided an effective and newly popular way to work out. Even the magazine *Men's Health*, which is geared to the young and fit, praised the approach for its ability to pack on muscle and predicted that these workouts would endure long after the pandemic receded.

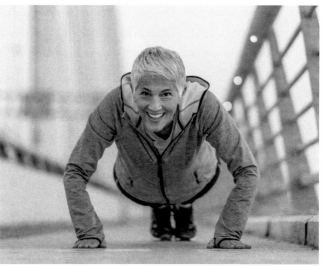

© liubaophoto | Getty Images

When you do a push-up—a classic body-weight exercise—you don't need any barbells or machines to strengthen not only your upper arms, but also your core.

But don't be intimidated by these tributes to the rigorous nature of body-weight exercise. As with many types of physical activity, the exercises themselves can range from easy to hard. This report allows you to adjust your workout to your level of ability. It also provides a well-rounded program, exercising all the major muscles and giving you a mix of strength training and cardio exercise.

The classic body-weight exercises are muscle-building moves that substitute your own body for the weight you would otherwise hoist. For example, when you do a push-up, there's not a barbell in sight, but you're still applying muscle strength to move a lot of pounds. Other typical body-weight exercises include squats and lunges, in which your leg muscles raise and lower your body, while your core muscles provide crucial stabilization. But body-weight training also includes cardio exercises, as long as your body is the driver of the motion. Examples include walking, running, and jumping jacks.

The beauty of body-weight exercise is that even short workouts can deliver results. The Royal Canadian Air Force created a five-exercise program that takes only 11 minutes to complete. In this report, you'll find two similar workouts, called 10-minute cardio interval workouts—one that features low-impact exercise and another that concentrates on high-impact moves. You'll also find strength and core workouts at two levels of difficulty, labeled "basic" and "challenge." And for variety, we've added a short balance workout and a 3-minute cardio workout you can do in spare moments of the day.

But first, here's some information to help you understand a bit about body mechanics and why body-weight exercise is so beneficial.

Gravity's gift

You are constantly working against gravity as you go about your daily life. Even when you're standing still, muscles throughout your body, the so-called antigravity muscles—from your legs (calf muscles, quadriceps, and gluteals) to your upper back (the erector spinae)—are working to keep you upright. But the more you move, the more energy you're expending to counter this unseen force.

To understand just how effective everyday weight-bearing exercise is, consider the experience of astronauts, who are weightless when they are in outer space. Research has found that astronauts can lose up to 20% of their muscle mass in less than two weeks when they are deprived of the resistance of gravity. That's because the body, in its wisdom, does not put its resources into maintaining muscles that have minimal demands placed on them. Even bone density declines at a rate of up to 10% in six months, when bones no longer have to harden themselves to withstand the forces of terrestrial life. To maintain muscle and bone mass while in outer space, astronauts have to exercise for two to two-and-a-half hours a day, using special equipment that provides resistance.

Unlike the astronauts in outer space, we on Earth have gravity to help us, day in and day out. But how much benefit you derive from it depends on how much you get up and move around. Failing to take advantage of it is like leaving dumbbells in the corner to gather dust or turning your treadmill into a clothes hanger.

Even doing a single exercise is better than doing nothing. For one study, a small group of frail 70-somethings were instructed to do 48 chair stands twice a week for 12 weeks. A chair stand (page 26) is a simple exercise in which you stand up from a chair and sit down again repeatedly, using only your muscles to power the movement. It's a perfect example of body-weight exercise and is something you can easily do at home, even while watching TV. And it's surprisingly effective. During the 12 weeks of the study, the participants increased their muscle mass by about 6% (instead of seeing declines, which are typical at this age) and boosted the strength of their quadriceps (the muscles in the front of the thigh) by about 10%.

To derive the full benefits of gravity, try to meet the recommendations set out in the Physical Activity Guidelines for Americans from the U.S. Department of Health and Human Services (see "Exercise guidelines," page 15). They specifically mention body-weight exercise as one way to fulfill the recommendation for strength training.

The advantages of body-weight exercise

All exercise is beneficial. But even stacked up against other types of workouts, body-weight exercise has a lot to offer. Not only does it provide an excellent workout, but it can also help you overcome some common excuses for avoiding exercise, like "I don't have time to go to the gym" and "I don't have space for a stationary bike at home." All you have to do is move your body. And you don't have to worry about dropping a heavy dumbbell on your toes!

Here's a closer look at some of the pluses.

It couldn't be more convenient. No matter where you are, you've got your body, so you can start exercising anywhere, anytime—in your bedroom when you wake up, in the kitchen while you're waiting for water to boil, in your hotel room when traveling, at the park while watching your kids or grandkids play, in your office while working. That makes it easy to find the time. You don't need to spend half an hour driving to the gym and back. Instead, you can exercise right here, right now, even if you only have 15 minutes to spare.

The price is right. With body-weight exercise, there's nothing to buy other than a pair of shoes. You don't need stylish clothing. You don't even need a yoga mat, much less an expensive gym membership, although you can certainly do these workouts at the gym, too. And your body, unlike some exercise equipment, is never hard to get. You might want a few props, such as a chair, bench, or counter to modify some moves, but these are all items that you have on hand.

The intimidation factor is low. You can do these exercises solo. You don't have to walk into a gym full of buff exercisers and complicated-looking weight machines that require adjustments and may still not fit you properly. You don't have to try to figure out which weights or other pieces of equipment to buy, or worry about hoisting heavy, bulky dumbbells. It's just you—and you're already familiar with how your body works.

It's effective. The military and world-class gymnasts wouldn't use body-weight training if it didn't deliver results. Research published in the journal *Physiology and Behavior* found that, as a form of resistance training, body-weight exercise helps build muscle "independent of an external load." But it does more than that. When Polish researchers looked at the effects of 10 weeks of body-weight exercises on various physical fitness parameters in a small group of young women, they found improvements in seven out of nine of the parameters. The biggest gains were in aerobic capacity, with a 33% improvement. Muscle endurance, particularly in the core, increased by 11%, while lower-body power posted a 6% gain. Even flexibility was better after the training.

You don't necessarily have to do a lot of it. While it's good to meet the Physical Activity Guidelines, smaller amounts of body-weight exercise can also deliver results. In a small study of active people in their 60s, Japanese researchers found that a workout consisting of eight simple lower-body exercises—including squats, knee lifts, heel raises, and other exercises in this report—increased the participants' muscle strength and power by about 15% after 10 months. That may not sound like much, but during this stage of life, strength and power are often declining. What's more, the participants achieved these gains by doing only six workouts *a month*.

It provides "functional" exercise. Most body-weight exercises work multiple muscles at once rather than training an isolated muscle or muscle group, as many exercise machines and dumbbell exercises do. Therefore, body-weight exercises are considered more functional, using more muscles and joints at a time, engaging balance and proprioception (awareness of where your body is in space), and mimicking everyday activities like pushing open doors, climbing stairs, and picking things up off the floor. It's kind of like training for a sport, but the sport you're training for is real life.

It can be adjusted to your fitness level. It may not be obvious how to do this at first. When you're using your body as the weight, you can't just remove 10 or 20 pounds as you can with machines or dumbbells. But there are ways to modify moves to decrease or increase the resistance. You can adjust your body position—for example, doing push-ups against a wall rather than the floor—or you can change the number of times you repeat an exercise or modify the pace you're working at. The workouts in this report were designed to help with this by progressing from easier to harder and offering modifications to accommodate all levels.

It's good for your health. Literally thousands of studies have shown that the more you move, the lower your risks for heart disease, diabetes, obesity, multiple types of cancer, joint pain, and Alzheimer's disease. Exercise can also lift your mood, reduce your stress level, and improve your sleep.

Body-weight exercise is no exception. Here's one example: Researchers in Brazil recruited a small group of postmenopausal women whose blood sugar levels were in the prediabetic range, placing them at high risk for diabetes. The women were then assigned to either a body-weight training program or a traditional training program. The body-weight program consisted of 30-second intervals of step-ups (page 30) and squats (page 13) followed by 60 seconds of easy walking. This routine was repeated 10 times per session. The traditional group walked for 30 minutes and lifted weights. Both groups exercised three times a week. After 12 weeks, both groups had greater muscle mass and were walking faster, and they also showed significant improvements in risk factors for diabetes, according to findings reported in the journal *Menopause* in

2019. In fact, some of the women were no longer classified as prediabetic. And because the body-weight exercises were performed in high-intensity intervals, the workouts could be shorter while delivering similar gains. The cardio interval workouts in this report (pages 27, 37, and 50) will show you how to incorporate intervals into your exercise program.

Your body in action

Compared with exercise equipment in the gym, your body is vastly more complex and has a lot more moving parts. More than 200 bones, 600 skeletal muscles, and about 45 miles of nerves are behind the myriad of voluntary movements your body makes every day. It's the interplay of muscles and bones (musculoskeletal system) and nerves and muscles (neuromuscular system) that enables you to walk, jump, twist, reach, lift, and more.

Many muscles, one movement

Movement begins with the brain sending electrical signals down the spinal column and out through nerves to your muscles, causing them to contract. Then muscles pull on bones, generating force, to make the movement happen. But this involves more complicated coordination among muscles than many people realize.

Figure 1: Major skeletal muscles

With 600 skeletal muscles in your body, it would be difficult for most people without training in anatomy to identify them all. But it's worth knowing the names and locations of the major ones, such as the quadriceps and hamstrings. This illustration shows most of the major skeletal muscles. However, some important muscles are not visible here, since they are underneath other muscles. For example, the internal obliques lie underneath the external obliques. And hip flexors including the psoas major and minor lie deep beneath the lower portion of the rectus abdominis.

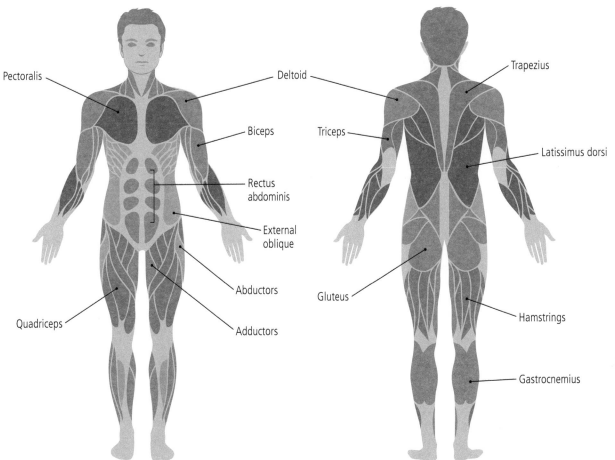

Muscles work in opposing pairs. As one contracts and pulls on a bone, the opposing muscle relaxes until it is its turn to contract and move the bone in the opposite direction. The muscle that delivers most of the force needed for a specific movement is called the agonist. The opposing muscle, which helps control the speed and force of the movement and prevent injury, is called the antagonist. So, as you walk up stairs, the quadriceps muscles on the fronts of your thighs act as agonists, while the hamstring muscles at the backs of your thighs work as antagonists, helping you move in a controlled and fluid way. This synergistic relationship is the reason you need to exercise both muscles; otherwise, you will create an imbalance in strength that can increase your chances of injury (see "Your body's kinetic chain," below left). That's why the strength workouts in this report work all the major muscle groups.

While it's clear that you need the major leg muscles in order to climb the stairs, they are not the only muscles your body recruits for that task. The body also uses muscles deep in your pelvis, such as the iliopsoas, to assist the quadriceps in the movement. These helper muscles are known as synergists, or secondary movers.

During any movement, there are also muscles that act as stabilizers to help keep you upright. For example, your abdominal and back muscles support your posture as you climb the stairs, so that you don't lose your balance and fall. Stabilizers work harder when you are standing than sitting, and even harder if you're climbing, working on an unstable surface, or balancing on one leg.

There are practical implications to this information, because you can use it to make an exercise easier or harder. For example, if you're sitting while performing an exercise, it will be easier than if you are standing. When you're standing with your feet apart, your stabilizers have an easier job than when your feet are together. To really challenge them, balance on one leg while you execute a move. This is just one example of how you can manipulate your body position to change an exercise's level of difficulty.

Three types of muscle contraction

Although it's common to think that muscles do nothing more than contract and relax, it's actually more complicated than that. Whether you're performing the exercises in this report or just moving throughout your day, your muscles will engage in three types of contractions. Paying attention to what your muscles are doing as you execute a move will improve your form and technique, so there's less chance of injury.

Your body's kinetic chain

One look at a skeleton tells you a lot about the human body. Every bone in it adjoins another bone, usually meeting end-to-end. Add in the muscles, ligaments, and tendons that hold this structure together and enable it to move, and you have an interconnected system, in which movement in one part can affect the others. This concept, known as the kinetic chain, was originally used in engineering and then later adapted to human movement and rehabilitation. What it teaches us is simple, but important: if there is misalignment or weakness in one area of the body, it tends to cause problems in others.

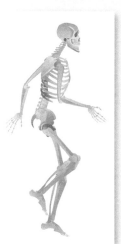

This is most obvious when you have an injury. For example, if you sprain your left ankle, you shift your weight more quickly than usual off the left foot when you walk, landing more heavily on the right. This combination of force and misalignment can trigger bursitis and pain in your right hip or knee. New problems can zigzag up the body, making you vulnerable to further injuries, particularly if muscles supporting the other joints are weak.

Less obviously, problems can arise if opposing sets of muscles are not equally strong. The knee is a prime example. For the kneecap to track properly, the muscles above and below it need to be balanced. If one muscle is stronger, tighter, or weaker than the others, your knee joint may not function properly. This may result in knee pain or in problems up or down the kinetic chain—in your back or hips, or in your foot or ankle.

Because your body functions as a unit, it's important that you exercise all the major muscles so imbalances don't develop. And it's also important to move in all the planes of motion—forward and back, side to side, and rotational—to preserve strength in some less frequently used muscles.

Concentric action occurs when muscles exert force and move joints while *shortening*. When people think of using their muscles, this is usually what comes to mind—for example, flexing an arm to show off the biceps muscle in the upper arm. This is the same type of motion you would use when bending your arms to lift a bag of groceries out of the back of the car or hoisting the bag up to the kitchen counter. When you do power training—a type of exercise that trains so-called fast-twitch muscle fibers (see "Two types of muscle fiber," page 8)—this is the part of the contraction that you speed up.

Eccentric action occurs when muscles exert force and move joints while *lengthening*. As you slowly lower your grocery bag, the biceps muscles lengthen while producing force, so that you lower the object in a controlled manner rather than simply letting it drop. Eccentric strength is especially important for balance, mobility, and everyday functions. Slowing down the eccentric phase of an exercise has been shown to improve strength gains. However, you are also more likely to experience soreness a day or so after training in this manner. The strength workouts in this report use tempos that achieve maximum strength gains with minimal soreness.

Isometric (static) action creates force, too, but the muscles don't shorten or lengthen much and joints do not move. If you push against a wall, for example, or try to lift an object that is far too heavy for you, you'll feel your arm muscles tense. But since your muscles can't generate enough force to lift the object or shift the wall, they stay in the same position instead of shortening. Your core muscles engage in a lot of iso-

How to avoid "dead butt syndrome"

There are many reasons to stand up and move around during the day rather than staying glued to your desk chair or a driver's seat. Habitual inactivity raises risks for more than 30 ailments, including obesity, diabetes, heart disease, and more. But here's one problem you may not have heard of. It's called gluteal amnesia—or as its more colorful moniker puts it, "dead butt syndrome."

It occurs when the gluteus medius—one of three gluteal muscles, which helps stabilize the pelvis and maintain your body's proper alignment—becomes too weak to do its job. This can happen in different ways, but one is simply lack of activity. When it's rarely called upon to contract, the gluteus medius lengthens. At the same time, the hip flexors in the front of your thighs tighten because they are constantly contracted when you're in a flexed (seated) position. This creates an imbalance between these two opposing muscle groups, so they don't work together as effectively. The result can be a smaller range of motion, plus pain or numbness in your buttocks. And when the gluteus medius isn't functioning properly, muscles above, below, and around it may be called on to pick up the slack, potentially leading to hip, back, or knee pain. Gluteal amnesia also minimizes the effectiveness of exercises like squats that rely on the gluteus medius for stabilization.

Fortunately, with the right moves, you can prevent this problem from occurring—or, if you already have it, you can bring the dysfunctional muscle back into working order. First, stand and move around more during the day. Second, expand your exercise repertoire to include exercises that emphasize side-to-side movement such as side lunges (page 19), clams (page 36), grapevines (page 29), side leg lifts (pages 25 and 49), side hops (page 38), and skaters (page 51). These will help to strengthen the gluteus medius and other lateral-working muscles. Third, don't forget to stretch after exercising. Stretches that target the hip area can be helpful. For example, the hip flexor stretch (page 41) helps lengthen the hip flexors.

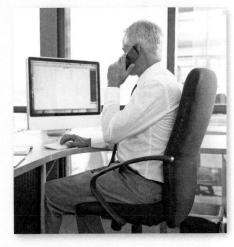

metric contractions to keep you standing tall. This is also the action of exercises like planks, where you hold a position (see "Kneeling plank," page 25).

Here's what all of that means in practical terms. Concentric and eccentric muscle actions create movement, whether you are lifting a suitcase, dancing, or simply walking across a room. As you perform an exercise, the muscle targeted by that exercise will alternate between concentric and eccentric actions. By contrast, your core muscles perform isometric contractions to maintain your stability and balance during all types of activities.

© shapecharge | Getty Images

Two types of muscle fiber

To produce various movements, skeletal muscles rely on two main types of muscle fibers, called slow-twitch and fast-twitch based on how quickly they contract. Each enables a different type of action.

Slow-twitch fibers do not tire easily and are in it for the long haul. These fibers power aerobic activities such as walking, biking, swimming, and jogging. Fast-twitch fibers produce bursts of speed, but they tire quickly. They provide the power for sprinting, jumping, or racing up a flight of stairs.

In practice, both types of fibers are often activated during everyday activities. For example, your slow-twitch fibers are firing while you're out walking your dog, but when you have to sprint after him at the dog park, those fast-twitch fibers kick in. Similarly, when you're cutting the grass, your slow-twitch fibers are running the show, until you have to move some big rocks out of the way. Then your fast-twitch fibers are recruited for a short, intense burst of power. That's why you need to train both types of fibers, and you do that in different ways.

Traditional strength training and low-impact cardio exercise typically train slow-twitch fibers. Power training, which adds a speed component to strength moves, targets the fast-twitch fibers. For example, you might lift your hips more quickly during a bridge (page 21) or press up more quickly during a push-up (pages 22 and 31). Jumping exercises (plyometrics) are a type of cardio exercise that targets fast-twitch fibers. Many workout programs overlook power training, but it's an important component to ensure you stay active and at your best for many years to come.

Three planes of motion

Challenging your muscles in multiple ways is important. Training both slow-twitch and fast-twitch fibers is a good start, but you also need to move in different directions. The body has three planes of motion in which movement happens, and different muscles are activated depending upon the plane you are moving in.

Sagittal plane motion, the most common, is forward and backward—for example, walking to the mailbox or going out for a run or bike ride. The primary movers for these movements are the large muscles in your legs (quadriceps, hamstrings, and calf muscles) and buttocks (gluteus maximus).

Frontal plane motion is lateral—for instance, navigating obstacles in your path or doing grapevine steps in an exercise class. For these movements, you're recruiting muscles on the outer portions of your legs and hips (such as the gluteus medius, gluteus minimus, and tensor fascia latae).

Transverse plane motion is rotation. Twisting while driving to look over your shoulder and swinging a golf club or tennis racquet are examples of this type of movement. These movements rely on the abdominal muscles that wrap around your torso (internal and external obliques).

The more you move in a given direction, the stronger and more adept at certain movements those muscles become. But when you're not moving as often in a particular plane of motion, those muscles can become weaker and create imbalances that affect your body's kinetic chain (see page 6), possibly resulting in injuries. That's why it's important to train in all planes of motion—for example, squats (pages 20 and 32) in the sagittal plane, side lunges (page 28) in the frontal plane, and twists (page 42) in the transverse plane. If you do a strength, core, and cardio workout, as we recommend, you get all three.

You can even add movement in a different plane of motion to increase the difficulty of an exercise and work more muscles. For example, add a twist to the stationary lunge (page 31) to work in both the sagittal and transverse planes. Or add a lateral move to the half squat (page 20) by stepping out to the side as you lower into the squat, then bringing your feet back together as you stand up. Now you're training in both the sagittal and frontal planes. Some moves, like the squat with knee lift and rotation (page 34), involve all three planes of motion. ♥

Safety first

In general, moderate activity is safe for most people. Still, everything you do, even getting out of bed or stepping into your bathtub, carries some risk, so it's wise to review basic safety guidelines before starting a new exercise program. This chapter covers common issues, like whether you need to consult a doctor before starting and what precautions you should take if you have certain conditions, such as heart disease or arthritis. It also includes safety tips that are useful for everyone, no matter how young and fit. And it provides pointers on maintaining good form, which can help you prevent injuries.

When to see a doctor

Never hesitate to talk to your doctor about your exercise goals and plans. Besides yourself, your doctor is in the best position to evaluate your abilities and recommend modifications if necessary. In fact, having his or her support may even help to keep you motivated.

You will definitely need to talk to your doctor before starting an exercise program if you're a smoker or have quit within the past six months, or if you have any injuries or an unstable chronic health condition, including

- heart disease (or multiple risk factors for it)
- diabetes
- a respiratory ailment, such as asthma
- high blood pressure
- joint or bone disease such as osteoarthritis or osteoporosis
- musculoskeletal problems such as knee, shoulder, or back issues, including herniated discs
- a stroke or neurologic illness
- a joint replacement
- a recent surgery
- medication that can make you dizzy or lightheaded.

A helpful resource for gauging your ability is the Get Active Questionnaire from the Canadian Society for Exercise Physiologists. You can find it online at www.health.harvard.edu/GAQ.

If you do need to speak to a doctor, bring, fax, or email descriptions of the exercises in this report that you plan to do, and ask if you can safely undertake them. Your doctor may feel your selections are fine or might wish to modify certain moves or suggest substitutions.

If necessary, your doctor can refer you to a physiatrist (a physician who specializes in physical medicine and rehabilitation), a physical therapist, or another specialist for evaluation. These professionals can tailor an exercise prescription to your specific needs if you're recovering from surgery or injuries, or if you have chronic problems that interfere with exercise by sparking pain or limiting movements. They can also tell you whether certain types of exercises will be helpful or harmful given your situation. Usually, you'll be able to find a safe, enjoyable selection, though some precautions may be in order. Following are some safety tips for people with various chronic conditions.

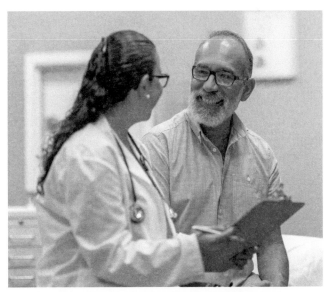

Moderate activity is safe for most people. But you should consult a doctor if you have chronic health problems or recently had surgery. Your doctor can help you modify exercises, if necessary.

Tips for people with specific conditions

If you have heart disease, diabetes, arthritis, or osteoporosis, it is imperative that you speak with your doctor before you start any exercise program. Once your physician has signed off on your exercise plans, the following tips may help you get more out of your workouts and avoid injury.

If you have heart disease

- Don't hold your breath while performing resistance exercises. Holding your breath while straining to execute a move can raise blood pressure dangerously. Counting out loud as you perform a move will prevent you from holding your breath.
- Don't push through fatigue, which can be a signal that you're overdoing it. If you feel tired or have any heart symptoms (see "Warning signs," below right), stop.
- Be aware that many drugs given to help treat heart disease may affect you when you're exercising. Beta blockers, for example, keep heart rate artificially low; that means your pulse is not a good indicator of how vigorously you are exercising. Vasodilators and ACE inhibitors may make you more prone to dizziness from a drop in blood pressure if your post-exercise cool-down is too short. Talk with your doctor about the medications you take and how they may affect the exercises you are planning to perform.

If you have diabetes

- Talk with your doctor about adjusting your medications before you start or ramp up an exercise program. Exercise requires glucose, so it may affect the dose of medication you need and maybe even the timing of your doses.
- Schedule eating and exercise sessions to keep blood sugar levels steady. In general, the best time to exercise is one to three hours after eating, when your blood sugar level is likely to be higher.
- Keep quickly digested carbohydrates, such as hard candy or glucose tablets, with you when you exercise in case your blood sugar drops precipitously, a condition called hypoglycemia. Signs of hypoglycemia include sweating, trembling, dizziness, hunger, and confusion.
- Wear a diabetes bracelet or ID tag and carry phone numbers of your emergency contacts in case of an emergency while you're exercising.

If you have arthritis

- Schedule workouts for times of the day when your medications are working well, in order to reduce inflammation and pain. For example, avoid morning workouts if stiffness is at its worst then.
- Before you exercise, apply heat to sore joints or take a warm shower or bath to ease stiffness. After exercise, cold packs may be helpful to minimize inflammation.
- If you have rheumatoid arthritis or another form of inflammatory arthritis, include some gentle stretching after you warm up. Inflammation weakens the tendons that tie muscle to bone, making them more susceptible to injury. Remember to use slow movements during your warm-up, and gradually extend your range of motion.
- If you have rheumatoid arthritis, add more rest

> **Warning signs**
>
> **Signs of an emergency.** If you experience any of these symptoms during or after exercise, call 911:
>
> ✔ upper-body discomfort, including chest pain, aching, burning, tightness, or a feeling of uncomfortable fullness
>
> ✔ significant or persistent wheezing, shortness of breath, or dizziness that takes longer than five minutes to go away
>
> ✔ faintness or loss of consciousness.
>
> These warning signs pertain to any kind of exercise—strength training and aerobic exercise alike.
>
> **Signs that should prompt a call for advice.** Persistent or intense muscle pain that starts during a workout or right afterward, or muscle soreness that lasts more than one to two weeks, also merits a call to your doctor. (This is in contrast to normal muscle soreness, which starts 12 to 48 hours after a workout and gradually improves.) You should also call your doctor if the routine you've been doing for a while without discomfort starts to cause you pain.

time to your routine when your condition flares up to reduce inflammation, pain, and fatigue. When it calms down, you can exercise more. Staying active with frequent rest breaks tends to help more than long periods spent in bed.

- Exercise within a comfortable range of motion. If an exercise causes significant pain, stop doing it! Discuss other options with your trainer or physical therapist.

Generally, water workouts or walking may be a better choice than higher-intensity or higher-impact activities.

If you have osteoporosis

- Protect your spine. Avoid activities and exercises that require you to bend or twist your spine.
- Avoid jumping and other high-impact activities.

Posture and alignment check

Posture counts a lot when you're exercising. Aligning your body properly is the key to good form, which nets you greater gains in fitness, while helping you avoid injuries. In fact, good posture and body alignment help anytime you're moving. If one foot is always turned slightly inward, for example, it impedes the power of your movement whether you're walking, going up stairs, jogging, or playing sports. If your heels come off the floor when you perform squats, it puts excessive stress on your ankle joints. And because each bone in your body is linked to the next one (see "Your body's kinetic chain," page 6), the effects of misalignments like these can zigzag their way up your body, paving the way for injuries to the ankle, knee, hip, and beyond.

Quick posture checks before and during exercise ensure that all parts of your kinetic chain are in alignment to help you avoid injury and squeeze the most benefit from your workout. If possible, look in a mirror when you do each exercise until you get the hang of it. This enables you to observe your body position and correct sloppy form. Try to take a few moments each day to practice better posture, too.

When exercise instructions in our workouts ask you to stand up straight, that means the following:

- Your chin is parallel to the floor.
- Both shoulders are even and back and down.
- Your ears are aligned with your shoulders.
- Both hips are even.
- Your shoulders are aligned with your hips.
- Abdominal muscles are actively working.
- Your hips are aligned with your knees.
- Both knees are even and pointed straight ahead.
- Your knees are aligned with your ankles.
- Both feet are pointed straight ahead.
- Body weight is evenly distributed on both feet.

In addition, it's important to maintain a neutral spine. A neutral spine takes into account the slight natural curves of the spine, but it's not flexed or arched. One way to find the neutral position is to lift your tailbone as far as is comfortable to arch your lower back, then tuck your tailbone under to flatten your lower back. The spot approximately in the middle should be neutral. If you're not used to standing or sitting up straight, it may take a while for this to feel natural. When you are instructed to bend, do so at the hips, not at the waist, and keep your spine neutral and your core muscles contracted to protect your back.

Few of us have perfect posture, which is why it's so important to check your posture before and during each exercise. Each exercise in our workouts includes tips on good technique, so make sure you review them before trying the move.

Paying attention as you perform upper-body exercises may also alert you to muscle imbalances based on whether your right or left side is dominant. If you notice this, focus on your weaker side to make sure it's not slacking off. Over time, this will help to even out the imbalance and give you a better workout.

Tips for safe exercise

Exercise is so good for you, doctors are starting to write prescriptions for it. However, it's important to follow certain safety guidelines.

All-around exercise safety tips

Whatever kind of exercise you choose to do, following these general tips can help you protect yourself from injury and maximize benefits.

Warm up properly. In general, you should allot five to 10 minutes to warm up before a workout. This allows your body to prepare for exercise by providing more oxygen to your muscles, lubricating your joints, and increasing your range of motion.

Pay attention to your body. Don't exercise when you're sick or feeling overly fatigued. Fatigue often leads to injuries.

Don't overdo it. Unless you already exercise frequently and vigorously, plan to work your way up to high-intensity activities over time. Going too hard or doing too much too soon can cause overuse injuries like stress fractures, stiff or sore joints and muscles, and inflamed tendons and ligaments.

Respect the weather. When humidity is high or the thermometer is expected to reach 80° F or higher, exercise during cooler morning or evening hours or in an air-conditioned space. When exercising outside in cold weather, dress in layers, including gloves and hat. If you have asthma or another respiratory problem, plan to exercise indoors when air quality is especially unhealthy. Seasonal allergy sufferers benefit from moving indoors, too, when pollen counts are high or other allergens abound.

Stay hydrated. Drink sufficient fluids throughout the day and while exercising, especially if it's hot or humid. Proper hydration will keep your muscles functioning at a high level and help to prevent headaches and fatigue.

Watch for signs of overheating. In hot, humid weather, be aware that a headache, dizziness, nausea, faintness, cramps, or palpitations could all be signs of overheating. If you notice any of these symptoms, stop exercising, get out of the heat, and rehydrate.

Don't forget to cool down and stretch afterward. Gradually slow your activity at the end of a workout. Stopping abruptly can leave you feeling lightheaded or dizzy, which could lead to a fall. Finishing off with some stretches after your cool-down will improve your flexibility and range of motion.

Allow time for rest and recovery. Don't attempt high-intensity or high-impact workouts every day of the week. Instead, allow a rest day (which might include low- or moderate-intensity activity to ensure that you get at least five days of exercise in a week) between vig-

orous workouts to avoid burnout and injuries (see "My action plan," page 46).

Know when to dial back. Decrease the intensity of your workout if you are having difficulty finishing an exercise session, can't talk while exercising, or feel fatigued for the rest of the day after a workout. If you feel sick, hold off on exercise entirely until you feel well again for at least 24 hours.

Ease back in. If you stop exercising for a while, drop back to a lower level of exercise when you get started again and gradually build back up. For example, shorten your workouts or exercise at a lower intensity. Each week, increase your frequency, duration, or intensity a little more until you're back to your pre-hiatus routine. (Don't increase all of them at the same time, though.)

Strength training safety tips

When doing strength training, including the workouts in this report, follow these tips to help prevent injury.

Build up gradually. Strength is built by working a muscle against resistance like your body weight. But trying to do too much too soon can lead to injuries. This report offers two different workout levels, along with modifications to make exercises easier or harder. Start with the easiest and progress from there. It's safer to start with a workout that might be too easy for you; you can always try the more challenging options the next time. But if you start too hard and get injured, you could end up sidelined for days or even weeks.

Focus on form. Good form will ensure that you are getting the most benefits from an exercise and help you to avoid injuries. For example, when you do a lunge or a squat, you should never allow your knees to extend farther forward than the ends of your toes; going beyond that point can strain your knees (see "The right [and wrong] way to do two classic body-weight exercises," page 13). Throughout this report, we include instructions and tips to help you maintain good form. Also remember to follow the guidelines on posture (see "Posture and alignment check," page 11).

Don't lock your joints. Always leave a slight bend in your knees and elbows when straightening out your legs and arms. Hyperextended joints can strain ligaments around the joint.

The right (and wrong) way to do two classic body-weight exercises

Good form is crucial to protecting yourself from injury and getting the most benefit from an exercise. Here's a look at the right and wrong way to perform two exercises that are fundamental to a good body-weight workout.

SQUATS: DOS AND DON'TS

- *Do* bend at your hips to work your gluteal muscles and maintain proper knee alignment.
- *Do* lean forward about 45° to maintain balance.
- *Do* keep your feet flat with your heels on the floor to minimize stress on your ankle joints.
- *Don't* let your knees go farther forward than your toes. This will avoid putting excess pressure on the knee and ankle joints.
- *Don't* allow your knees to roll inward or outward as you squat. This will help you maintain proper alignment from your hips to your knees and on down to your ankles, to help avoid joint injuries.
- *Don't* round your back. This protects your spine from excess compression.

- *Don't* go lower than the point where your thighs are parallel to the floor. Sinking below this level is an important cause of knee injuries.

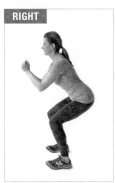 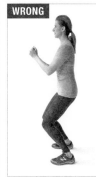 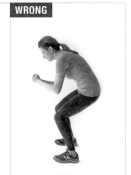

LUNGES: DOS AND DON'TS

- *Do* keep your front knee over your ankle to reduce pressure on your knee joint.
- *Do* keep your front knee in line with your toes so it's not pointing inward or outward, to avoid stressing your ankle and hip joints.
- *Do* keep your ears over your shoulders, your shoulders over your hips, and your hips over your back knee when you are in the down position. Proper alignment reduces pressure on joints and targets the muscles in your thighs and buttocks more effectively.
- *Do* keep your back knee pointing straight down toward the floor to avoid strain on your knee, hip, and ankle joints.
- *Don't* lean back, allowing your shoulders to lose alignment with the hips and fall backward, as this puts excess pressure on joints.

- Don't lean forward, as this puts excess pressure on your knee joints.
- Don't let your back heel roll outward or inward. It should be directly over your toes to avoid twisting your ankle or knees and increasing pressure on these joints.

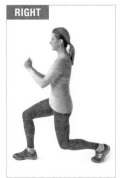 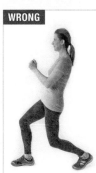 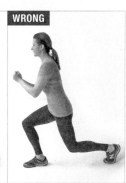

Work in a pain-free range of motion. When moving your arms or legs, stick with a range that feels comfortable. These exercises should not cause pain while you are doing them. Over time, gradually extend your range of motion through exercise and stretching.

Tempo, tempo. Work evenly at the pace specified in each exercise. Control is very important. Counting off the tempo aloud helps you stay in control, which enhances gains and helps you avoid injuries. It also ensures that you're not holding your breath.

Breathe. Blood pressure rises if you hold your breath during resistance exercises. Exhale as you work against gravity by lifting, pushing, or pulling; inhale as you release. During warm-ups and stretches, breathe comfortably.

Be smooth. Keep your movements slow and controlled. Jerky actions can lead to spraining or straining a muscle, tendon, or ligament.

Concentrate on the muscles you are working. In a study from Denmark, participants increased

If you injure yourself...

If you injure yourself in spite of your best efforts to keep safe, remember RICE—rest, ice, compression, and elevation.

Rest. Take the pressure off the injured area by reducing your activity and sitting or lying down.

Ice. To reduce inflammation, apply ice for 20 to 30 minutes every two to three hours during the first two or three days. Never apply ice directly to the skin. Wrap it in a towel, or use an ice pack or chemical cold pack.

Compression. Wrap an elastic bandage around the injured area to provide support and reduce swelling.

Elevation. To reduce inflammation and pain, prop the injured area on a pillow or on the arm of a sofa—anywhere it will be raised above waist level.

muscle activity up to 35% when they thought about the muscles they were working as they performed an exercise. The more muscle activity, the better results you'll get. To do this, bring your full attention to the muscles you are using during the exercise. Envision where they are in your body. Notice them contracting and relaxing.

Give muscles time off. As long as your muscles aren't sore, you could reasonably strength train on consecutive days. However, since the American College of Sports Medicine recommends only two or three complete strength workouts a week, consider giving yourself a day off in between. This will give your muscles time to recover, so they're fresh for the next workout.

Jumping safety tips

Here are some tips to maximize your efforts while minimizing your risk for injury when doing high-impact moves in the challenge-level 10-Minute Cardio Interval Workout (page 37) and the 3-Minute Cardio Interval Workout (page 50).

Wear supportive athletic shoes. Don't jump barefoot.

Choose a surface with some "give." Do not jump on hard surfaces like tile, concrete, or asphalt. These have no give in them and can lead to shin splints. Instead, choose a surface that can absorb some of the impact, such as a well-padded, carpeted wood floor indoors, or a level, smooth lawn outside.

Start slow and low. The faster you jump, the more intense the workout. So take your time when starting out. And aim for just a few inches off the floor. The higher you jump, the greater your impact on landing.

Land softly. Your toes and the balls of your feet should make the first contact with the ground, and then your weight sinks evenly down through your midfoot and into your heels. Bend your ankles, knees, and hips, leaning forward slightly to absorb some of the impact. Don't let your knees roll in toward each other as you land. Keep your knees over your feet.

Engage your core muscles. It's essential to protect your spine.

Stretching safety tips

Using proper technique for stretching can protect your muscles and joints.

Wait to stretch. At one time, stretching was considered a warm-up to exercise, but now we know better. Much like taffy, muscles stretch more easily when warm. That's why stretching after you work out is best for improving flexibility and increasing range of motion.

Feel no pain. Stretch only to the point of mild tension, never to the point of pain. You should feel the tension in the muscles, not in your joints. If a stretch hurts, stop immediately! Reset your position carefully and try again. With time and practice, your flexibility will improve.

Don't bounce. It's tempting to move deeper into a stretch by bouncing. However, that can injure muscles if the movements are not carefully controlled. Sudden movements trigger the so-called stretch reflex, which causes a lengthening muscle to shorten. Instead, move slowly. If you try to quickly touch your toes, you may not be able to do it, but if you reach toward your toes as far as is comfortable and just hang there for 15 to 30 seconds, your muscles will slowly lengthen, enabling you to get closer to your target.

Practice often. You'll see the best gains if you stretch frequently—several times a day on as many days of the week as possible. ◆

Program overview

The main workouts in this report are divided into two levels—basic and challenge. The basic level is for people who are just starting out or are getting back to working out regularly. The challenge level is for those who have some exercise experience. Within each level, you'll find a strength workout, a core workout, and a cardio interval workout. Once you've mastered these routines, you can add a little variety with the bonus workouts, starting on page 48.

Depending upon your fitness level, you can do all of the workouts in one level or choose from a combination of levels. For example, if you're an avid jogger but new to strength training, you might start with the basic-level strength and core workouts, but combine those with the challenge-level cardio interval workout.

If you're not sure where to start, go with the basic workouts to ensure you don't overdo it. You can always try something more difficult the next time. You'll also find modifications within each exercise to make it easier or harder. Listen to your body, and build the program that is right for you. Remember to warm up before working out, and cool down and stretch afterward. You'll find a warm-up routine on page 18 and stretches on page 40.

This chapter will show you how these workouts fit into formal exercise guidelines, give examples of how to adjust the challenge level of exercises, and explain the terminology used in the workout instructions.

Exercise guidelines

The Physical Activity Guidelines for Americans from the U.S. Department of Health and Human Services are a good place to start when creating an exercise plan. The guidelines recommend that all adults ages 18 to 64 include the following two types of exercise in their weekly routines:

- 150 to 300 minutes of moderate aerobic exercise per week—or 75 to 150 minutes of vigorous aerobic

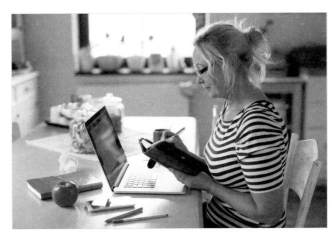

When you're having a busy day, it's easy to let exercise slide. One technique for making sure you actually do it is to schedule it on your calendar like any other appointment you need to keep.

exercise (see "Gauge your intensity," page 16). An equivalent mix of the two also works.
- two or more strength training sessions that target all of the major muscle groups per week.

People ages 65 and older should do as much as they can. Balance exercises (see "Balance Workout," page 48) are also recommended to help prevent falls. And routine activity during the day is also highly recommended. As the guidelines put it, "Move more and sit less."

You can use the cardio interval workouts in this report to help you fulfill the aerobic exercise recommendation. Since they are higher-intensity routines, you should mix in some moderate-intensity cardio activities like walking, swimming, or cycling for a well-rounded, balanced plan.

The strength workouts are total-body routines, so they will satisfy the strength recommendation. The core workouts also count toward the strength recommendation, but since they don't target all of the major muscle groups, you'll need to combine those with the strength workouts to meet the guidelines.

In addition to the main workouts, there are two supplementary workouts. The Balance Workout (page 48) is a good add-on to the main routine. If you're pressed for time or need an energy boost, try the 3-Minute Cardio Interval Workout (page 50). Mixing up your workouts will provide new challenges for your body so you keep getting results, and the variety will keep your workouts more interesting.

Adjusting the challenge

When you start a new routine, there are certain changes you will notice—like having more energy, being able to lift things more easily, seeing some definition in your muscles, and maybe even losing some pounds or inches. And then there are the changes that you can't see—like making your bones stronger, lowering your blood pressure, and improving your body's ability to manage blood sugar.

But as your body becomes accustomed to a particular workout, the gains level off. That's why you need to keep increasing the challenge. With traditional exercise equipment, you can add heavier weights. For body-weight exercises, you obviously can't do that, but there are other strategies you can use to increase—or decrease—the difficulty of moves.

One way is by altering the position of your body. In a classic chest press exercise, you lie on your back and raise and lower weights above your chest. For most people, doing this exercise without dumbbells or a resistance band isn't difficult. However, you can make it a challenging exercise by rolling over onto your belly and pushing up into a plank position. Now, you are supporting most of your body weight on your palms and the balls of your feet as you resist gravity's force. Almost every muscle in your body is working to keep you in this position. This is an example of an isometric contraction (see "Three types of muscle contraction," page 6). You can then take it up another notch, if you want, by performing push-ups—one of the classic body-weight exercises. Throughout the workouts, you'll see suggestions for ways to change body position to make exercises easier or harder.

Subtler changes, like adjusting your hand or foot position, can also alter the difficulty of an exercise. To return to the example of push-ups, the placement of the hands affects which muscles are targeted, according to a study in the *Journal of Physical Therapy Science*. For example, when the hands are closer together than the standard shoulder-width positioning, the triceps muscles in the backs of the upper arms and the infraspinatus muscles in the shoulder joints are activated more. By contrast, when the hands are positioned wider than shoulder-width apart, a key back muscle (the serratus anterior) that stabilizes the shoulder blades and protects the shoulder joint works harder. So, by changing up your hand position when you do push-ups, you'll work more muscles.

Your body also works as a series of levers. A lever is a rigid bar that hinges from or rotates around a fixed point. Joints act as the fixed points. During a side leg lift (pages 25 and 49), your leg is a lever with your hip joint as the fixed point. The shorter a lever is, the easier it is to lift. So, if you keep your knee bent as you lift your leg, that's easier than lifting it while it is extended. To make an exercise harder, lengthen the lever—for instance, by raising your arms overhead when you perform a half squat (page 20) or stationary lunge (page 31), or by extending your legs when you do triceps dips (page 32). It's similar with a push-up. Your entire body is a lever hinging from your ankle joints. When you shorten the lever by doing push-ups from your knees, they are easier. You can also change the difficulty based on how much gravity is acting on a lever. For example, doing push-ups on the floor in a horizontal position is more difficult than doing them while leaning diagonally or standing vertically, with your hands on a counter or wall. The same goes for a side leg lift. You're working more against gravity when you're lying on the floor (see "Side leg lift," page 25) than if you do them standing (see "Standing side leg lift," page 49).

Here are three more ways to mix up your workouts for additional benefits:

▶ Gauge your intensity

There are various ways to determine how hard you are exercising. But this one, known informally as the "talk test," is simple and intuitive.

- If you can sing and do the activity, it is low-intensity.
- If you can talk but not sing, it is moderate-intensity.
- If you can't sing or talk, it is vigorous or high-intensity.

You can increase the difficulty of body-weight exercises by changing the timing—for example, speeding up the movement, holding it for longer, or resting less in between sets.

Speed up your movement. Using a faster tempo for the exertion portion of exercises will increase power and help to maintain or even rebuild fast-twitch muscle fibers, which are responsible for short bursts of activity. In the strength workouts, you'll see rep and tempo guidelines (see "Terms to know," at right) for turning strength training exercises into power training exercises. We recommend that you get familiar with the strength moves by doing them for about two to four weeks before trying the power variations. When you're ready to move on to the power versions, you can do the full workout as a power workout, alternating the power workout with the strength workout. Or, you can do some exercises within a given workout as power moves and some as strength exercises. Mixing it up provides the best conditioning. No matter how you're training, you should aim for two or three such workouts a week.

Hold longer. Muscles store energy when they contract, and then—like a spring—that energy helps them snap back to their original position. Holding an exercise longer before returning to the starting position lets some of that energy dissipate. Then, when you start to move again, your muscles have to work harder. You'll see this technique used in some of the "Make it harder" sections, but feel free to apply it to any exercises you're doing if you want to boost the intensity.

Rest less. You can get more cardio benefits by moving quickly from one exercise to another with little to no rest in between. So, instead of doing multiple sets of an exercise, do just one, and then immediately move on to the next exercise. When you've completed all of the exercises in a workout, repeat them for a second set, and then a third set if you're up for it. By keeping your body moving without breaks, you'll kick up your heart rate and breathing to boost your cardiorespiratory fitness—and burn more calories.

Terms to know

Each exercise in the workouts includes instructions on how to perform it properly, including the starting position, the movement, and tips and techniques for maintaining good form. We also use certain terms you'll need to know.

Repetitions (reps). Each time you perform the movement in an exercise, that's called a rep. If you cannot do all the reps at first, just do what you can, and then gradually increase reps as you improve. When you are training for strength, aim for eight to 12 reps. For power training, you'll do fewer reps—six to 10—but at a faster pace (see "Tempo," below).

Sets. One set is a specific number of repetitions. For example, eight to 12 reps often make a single set. Usually, we suggest doing one to three sets.

Tempo. This tells you the count for the key movements in an exercise. For example, 3–1–3 means lift to a count of three, hold for one count, then lower to a count of three. If there are only two numbers, such as 2–2, that means you don't hold, so it's a continuous movement. Exercises with more parts have more numbers, and some, like those in the challenge-level 10-Minute Cardio Interval Workout (page 37), have no number, meaning the exercise is one fluid movement.

Hold. While most exercises have a hold as part of the tempo, some exercises like planks and stretches list "Hold" instead, since that is the focus of these moves. This line tells you the number of seconds to hold each.

Rest. Resting between sets gives your muscles a chance to recharge and helps you maintain good form. Except during the warm-up and cool-down activities, we specify a range of time to rest. How much of this time you need will differ depending on your level of fitness and how intensely you are working out. The less you rest, the more cardio benefits you will get from a workout, but don't overdo it. Listen to your body and rest when you need to.

In addition, most sets of instructions offer options to "make it easier" or "make it harder." These variations modify the exercise to be less challenging (for beginners or those with health concerns) or to increase the difficulty (for more advanced exercisers).

Now it's time to start working out! ♥

Warm-up

Before starting any workout, you should take at least five minutes to prepare your body for increased activity and reduce your risk of injury. By moving your muscles through a full range of motion, the exercises in this short routine will warm up all your major muscle groups so they're more pliable, lubricate your joints so they move more freely, and pump more nutrient-rich, oxygenated blood to your working muscles to fuel them for better performance.

Instructions: Perform 10 reps of each exercise (on both sides when appropriate) at a slow, four-to-six-count tempo. Then repeat the series of exercises again at a faster, two-to-three-count tempo.

Tips and techniques: Keep these pointers in mind as you do this routine:

- Maintain a neutral neck (with your head in line with your spine).
- Engage your core muscles.
- Don't lock your knees or elbows; keep them slightly bent.
- Keep your shoulders down and back, away from your ears.
- Keep your knee no farther forward than your toes when lunging.

What you need: Nothing.

---

1 | Shoulder roll

This simple exercise lubricates your shoulder joints to prepare them for larger arm movements.

Starting position: Stand up straight with your feet shoulder-width apart and your arms at your sides, palms facing back.

Movement: Roll your shoulders up, back, and down, keeping your elbows slightly bent. This is one rep. Complete 10 reps, and then roll your shoulders in the opposite direction: up, forward, and down.

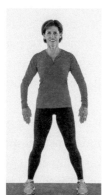 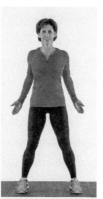

2 | Knee lift

A more dynamic version of marching in place, knee lifts start to warm up your lower body.

Starting position: Stand up straight with your feet together.

Movement: Lift your right knee as high as is comfortable, touching both hands to the knee. Lower your leg, and then repeat with your left knee. This is one rep.

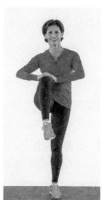 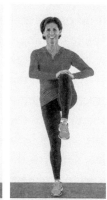

---

3 | Arm sweep

This exercise helps maintain range of motion in your shoulders, so reaching overhead is easier.

Starting position: Stand up straight with your feet together and your arms at your sides.

Movement: As you inhale, sweep your arms out to the sides and up toward the ceiling. As you exhale, sweep your arms back down to your sides. This is one rep.

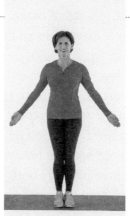 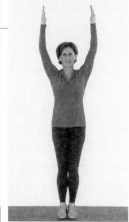

4 | High lunge

These lunges get your upper and lower body working together to improve coordination.

Starting position: Stand up straight with your feet wider than shoulder-width apart.

Movement: Rotate your torso to the left and reach with your right arm across your body as you shift your weight onto your left foot, bend your left knee, and tap your right foot out to the side. Return to the starting position and repeat, rotating to the right. This is one rep.

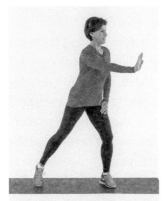 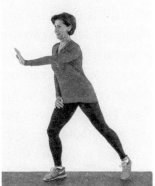

5 | Hamstring curl

Kick up your heart rate and pump more blood to power up your muscles.

Starting position: Stand up straight with your feet shoulder-width apart.

Movement: Bend your right knee, lifting your right foot behind you and bringing it toward your buttocks as you press your arms backward. Let your arms swing forward as you bring your leg back down. Repeat with your left leg. This is one rep.

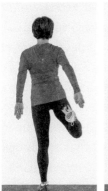 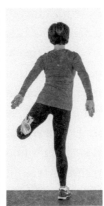

6 | Overhead reach

Stretch out the sides of your torso, an area often overlooked.

Starting position: Stand up straight with your feet shoulder-width apart and your arms at your sides.

Movement: Reach with your right arm up toward the ceiling, while shifting your weight to your left foot and tapping the toes of your right foot. Bring your left hand to your hip. Immediately repeat the move in the other direction, reaching up with your left arm as you shift your weight onto your right foot, tap your left foot, and bring your right hand down to your hip. This is one rep.

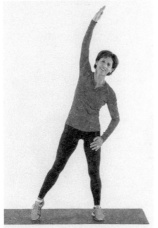 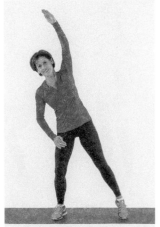

7 | Side lunge

Power up the muscles in your buttocks and legs.

Starting position: Stand up straight with your feet wider than hip width, toes pointing forward.

Movement: Bend your right knee, hinge forward at the hip, and bring both hands to your right thigh. Press into your right foot to stand up, and then repeat the lunge to the left. This is one rep.

Now, go back and repeat the entire sequence at a faster, two- to three-count tempo. 🛡

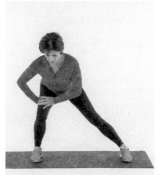 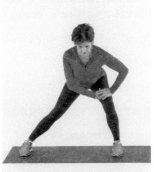

Basic level: Strength Workout

This workout targets all the major muscle groups with moves that exercise multiple muscles simultaneously to help keep your muscles and bones strong.

It can also help develop power, which is the product of both strength and speed. For example, strength may give you the ability to hike up a mountain trail, but power will help you react quickly if you trip over a root. It draws on fast-twitch fibers, as opposed to the slow-twitch fibers that are honed by classic strength training (see "Two types of muscle fiber," page 8). Power training may be even more important than strength training, because muscle power declines at twice the rate strength does as you age—as much as 3.5% a year for power compared with 1.5% for strength. The same exercises can develop both, if you just speed up part of the exercise, as indicated with the different tempos listed in each exercise.

Instructions: If you're not already warmed up when you start this workout, begin by performing the warm-up routine on page 18. Cool down afterward with three to five minutes of easy marching in place, and then wrap up by doing the stretches on page 40 to improve your flexibility and range of motion.

Aim to do this workout two or three times a week, preferably on nonconsecutive days. Beginners should follow the instructions for the standard form of each exercise for at least two weeks before moving on to the power variations or the "make it harder" options.

As noted, you can turn these strength exercises into power moves by using a faster tempo, as indicated below. Note that if you perform these as power exercises, you should reduce the number of reps, since the movement is harder. Therefore, you will see different numbers listed for both. If you want to derive cardio benefits from this workout, too, try reducing or eliminating the rest between sets and exercises.

What you need: Exercise mat or thick towel or carpet; sturdy chair.

---

1 | Half squat

This simple exercise will make it easier to get in and out of chairs or your car.

Starting position: Stand with your feet shoulder-width apart and your arms at your sides.

Movement: Slowly bend your hips and knees, lowering your buttocks about 8 inches, as if you're sitting back into a chair. Let your arms swing forward to help you balance. Keep your spine neutral. Hold. Slowly return to the starting position.

Reps: 8–12 for strength, 6–10 for power

Sets: 1–3

Tempo: 3–1–3 for strength, 3–1–1 for power

Rest: 30–90 seconds between sets

Tips and techniques:
- Shift your weight into your heels as you lower.
- Keep your abdominal muscles tight and your chest lifted.
- Don't let your bent knees extend beyond your toes.
- Tighten your buttocks as you stand to help you balance.

Make it easier: Sit on the edge of a chair with your feet hip-width apart and arms crossed over your chest. Tighten your abdominal muscles and stand up. Slowly sit down with control.

Make it harder: Lower your torso farther, but not past the point where your thighs are parallel to the floor. Place your hands behind your head or hold them overhead as you squat.

Harder

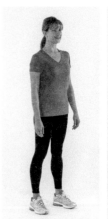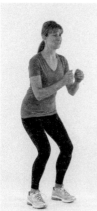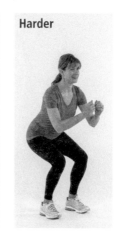

2 | Bridge

Bridges are one of the most effective core exercises, because they work multiple muscles on the back side of your body, from your upper back to your knees.

Starting position: Lie on your back with your knees bent and feet flat on the floor, hip-width apart and parallel to each other. Place your arms at your sides, palms up.

Movement: Tighten your buttocks, then lift your hips up off the floor as high as is comfortable. Keep your hips even and spine neutral. Hold. Return to the starting position.

Reps: 8–12 for strength, 6–10 for power

Sets: 1–3

Tempo: 3–1–3 for strength, 1–1–3 for power

Rest: 30–90 seconds between sets

Tips and techniques:

- Don't press your hands or arms against the floor to help you lift.
- Keep your shoulders, hips, knees, and feet evenly aligned.
- Keep your shoulders down and relaxed against the floor.

Make it easier: Lift your buttocks just slightly off the floor.

Make it harder: Extend one leg off the floor to do one-leg bridges.

Harder

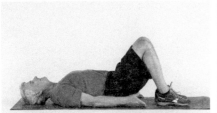
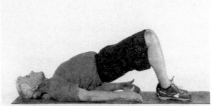
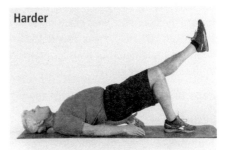

3 | Opposite arm and leg raise

This exercise—often used in physical therapy—challenges your balance and coordination while strengthening the muscles that run along your spine.

Starting position: Kneel on all fours with your hands and knees directly aligned under your shoulders and hips. Keep your head in line with your spine.

Movement: Extend your right leg off the floor behind you while reaching your left arm out in front of you. Try to raise your extended leg and arm parallel to the floor. Hold. Return to the starting position, then repeat with your left leg and right arm. This is one rep.

Reps: 8–12 for strength, 6–10 for power

Sets: 1–3

Tempo: 3–1–3 for strength, 1–1–3 for power

Rest: 30–90 seconds between sets

Tips and techniques:

- Keep your shoulders and hips level to maintain alignment throughout.
- Keep your head and spine neutral.
- Think of pulling your hand and leg in opposite directions, lengthening your torso.

Make it easier: Lift only your arm for eight to 12 reps, then lift only your leg for eight to 12 reps. Repeat on the other side.

Make it harder: Do all reps on each side without touching your hand and knee to the floor between reps.

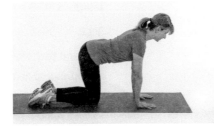
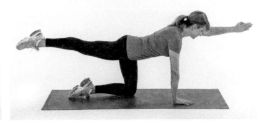

Easier

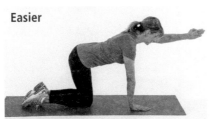

Easier

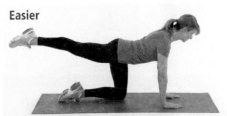

4 | Kneeling push-up

Push-ups are practically a total-body strengthener. For people who find push-ups too challenging, this modified version makes them more accessible.

Starting position: Kneel on all fours with your hands shoulder-width apart. Walk your hands forward and lower your hips so your body is at a 45° angle to the floor and forms a straight line from head to knees.

Movement: Bending your elbows out to the sides, slowly lower your upper body toward the floor until your elbows are bent about 90°. Hold. Press against the floor and straighten your arms to return to the starting position.

Reps: 8–12 for strength, 6–10 for power

Sets: 1–3

Tempo: 3–1–3 for strength, 3–1–1 for power

Rest: 30–90 seconds between sets

Tips and techniques:

• Keep your head in line with your spine.

• Keep your core muscles tight to prevent your back from arching too much.

• Don't bend at the hips.

• You can move your hands closer together or farther apart to work different muscles (see "Adjusting the challenge," page 16).

Make it easier: Stand up and do push-ups with your hands against a wall or a countertop.

Make it harder: Lift your knees off the floor and do push-ups, supporting yourself on your hands and the toes and balls of your feet. If that's too challenging, keep your feet on the floor and raise your hands by placing them on a chair seat, low bench, or step.

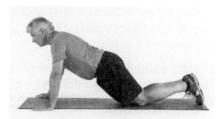

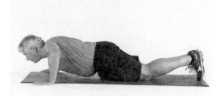

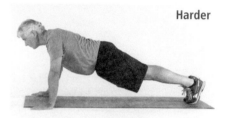

Harder

5 | Heel raise

This exercise, which you can do almost anywhere, builds well-defined calves—key anti-gravity muscles that keep you standing tall.

Starting position: Stand up straight behind a chair. Lightly hold on to the back of the chair with one or both hands, depending upon your need. Position your feet hip-width apart and evenly distribute your weight on both feet.

Movement: Tighten your abdominal muscles. Lift your heels off the floor, rising up onto your toes and balls of your feet. Hold. Slowly lower your heels to the floor, maintaining good posture as you do.

Reps: 8–12 for strength, 6–10 for power

Sets: 1–2

Tempo: 3–1–3 for strength, 1–1–3 for power

Rest: 30–90 seconds between sets

Tips and techniques:

• Keep your abdominal muscles tight.

• Keep your spine neutral and your shoulders down and back.

• Don't allow your ankles to roll inward or outward.

Make it easier: Don't lift your heels as high.

Make it harder: Balance on one foot and do one-leg heel raises.

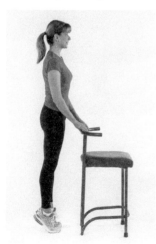

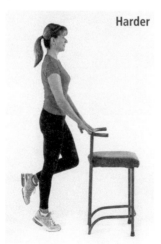

Harder

6 | Kneeling side plank

Side planks work key posture muscles on the sides of your body, which are often overlooked.

Starting position: Lie on your right side with your legs bent so your feet are behind you. Support your upper body on your right forearm with your shoulder aligned directly over your elbow. Place your left hand on your hip.

Movement: Tighten your abdominal muscles. Slowly lift your right hip and right thigh off the floor. Keeping your shoulders and hips stacked vertically, balance on your right forearm and the side of your right knee. Hold. Return to the starting position. If you held for less than 60 seconds, repeat. For example, if you can hold a plank for 15 seconds, you would do four reps. Then repeat on the other side.

Reps: as many as needed to hold for a total of 60 seconds on each side

Sets: 1

Hold: as long as possible, up to 60 seconds

Rest: 30–90 seconds between reps

Tips and techniques:

- Imagine your body is between two panes of glass; don't let your shoulders, hips, or head lean forward or back.
- Focus on lifting the bottom hip.
- Keep your shoulders down and back.

Make it easier: Hold for less than a total of 60 seconds.

Make it harder: Raise your top arm up toward the ceiling. ⬇

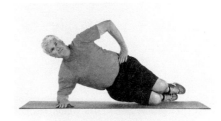

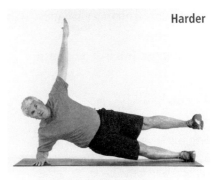

Harder

Basic level: Core Workout

Your core is much more than your abs. It also includes muscles in your back, sides, pelvis, hips, and buttocks. And this workout targets all of them. As the central link between your upper and lower body, a strong core enhances balance, stability, and efficiency of movement.

Instructions: If you're not already warmed up, begin by performing the warm-up routine on page 18. Finish your workout by doing the stretches on page 40 to improve your flexibility and range of motion.

Aim to do this workout two or three times a week, preferably on nonconsecutive days.

What you need: Exercise mat or thick towel or carpet; sturdy chair.

---

1 | Pelvic tilt

The movement here is small, but it can help you learn to engage your deep abdominal muscles, which will help you support your lower back.

Starting position: Lie on your back with your knees bent and feet flat on the floor, hip-width apart. Place your arms at your sides.

Movement: Exhale and gently tighten your abdominal muscles as if pulling your navel toward your spine, and slightly tilt your pelvis, flattening your lower back on the floor. Hold. Return to the starting position.

Reps: 8–12

Sets: 1–3

Tempo: 2–2–2

Rest: 30–90 seconds between sets

Tips and techniques:
- Because the movement is so subtle, try it once with your hands on your pelvis so you feel the pelvic tilt as you do it.
- Keep your shoulders down and back, relaxing them against the floor.
- Breathe comfortably even when you're holding the contraction.

Make it easier: Do fewer reps.

Make it harder: Hold the contraction for three to five counts before releasing.

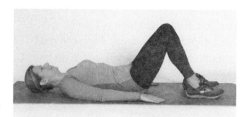
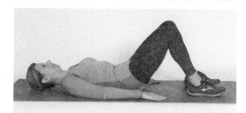

---

2 | Abdominal contraction

Once you've mastered the move, you can practice this core-strengthening exercise throughout the day, while sitting or standing.

Starting position: Kneel on all fours with your hands and knees directly aligned under your shoulders and hips. Keep your head and spine neutral.

Movement: Exhale as you tighten your abdominal muscles by pulling them up toward your spine. Keep your spine neutral. Hold. Release your abdominal muscles and return to the starting position.

Reps: 8–12

Sets: 1–3

Tempo: 2–2–2

Rest: 30–90 seconds between sets

Tips and techniques:
- This is a very subtle movement, and your spine should stay still throughout the exercise.
- Don't tilt your pelvis.
- Breathe comfortably even when you're holding the contraction.

Make it easier: Do fewer reps.

Make it harder: Hold the contraction for three to five counts before releasing.

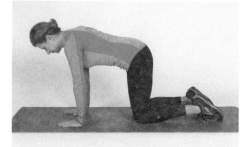

3 | Side leg lift

À la Jane Fonda, these leg lifts target the gluteus medius, one of the hip muscles. Weakness there can impair walking and contribute to knee pain.

Starting position: Lie on your right side with both legs extended and your head resting on your right arm. Place your left hand on the floor in front of you. Align your shoulders and hips evenly and keep your spine neutral.

Movement: Tighten your abdominal muscles. Raise your left leg toward the ceiling, keeping your hips stacked and facing forward. Hold. Return to the starting position. Finish all reps, then repeat on the other side. This completes one set.

Reps: 8–12 on each side

Sets: 1–3

Tempo: 2–1–2

Rest: 30–90 seconds between sets

Tips and techniques:

- Don't roll back onto your buttocks; stay on your hip.
- Don't let the knee of your lifting leg point up toward the ceiling; keep it pointing forward.
- Keep your shoulders and hips stacked vertically.
- Tighten your buttocks as you lift your leg.

Make it easier: Don't lift your leg as high. Or, bend your knee and lift your leg in that position.

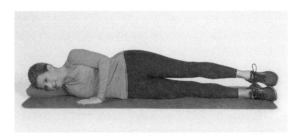
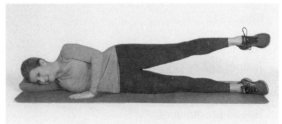

Make it harder: Hold your leg in the raised position for two to four counts before lowering it.

4 | Kneeling plank

Although planks involve no movement, supporting your body in a plank engages muscles throughout most of your body.

Starting position: Kneel on all fours with your hands and knees directly aligned under your shoulders and hips.

Movement: Tighten your abdominal muscles and walk your hands forward. Lower your upper body onto your forearms and drop your hips, so your body is in line from your head to your knees. Clasp your hands and align your shoulders directly over your elbows. Hold. If you held for less than 60 seconds, repeat. For example, if you can hold a plank for 15 seconds, you would do four reps.

Reps: as many as needed to hold for a total of 60 seconds

Sets: 1

Hold: as long as possible, up to 60 seconds

Rest: 30–90 seconds between reps

Tips and techniques:

- Keep your neck and spine neutral during the plank.
- Keep your shoulders down and back.
- Don't bend at your hips.

Make it easier: Do a plank standing up with your arms on a desk or counter.

Make it harder: Extend your legs, so your body is in a straight line, and hold the plank while balancing on your toes and balls of your feet.

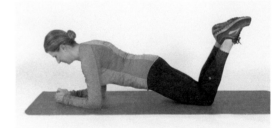
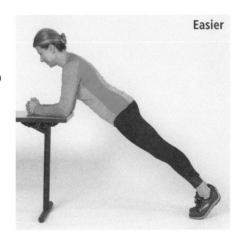

Easier

5 | Chair stand

Every time you get out of a chair you're doing this move, which makes it a functional exercise (one that prepares your body for everyday activities).

Starting position: Sit in a chair with your feet hip-width apart. Place your hands on your thighs.

Movement: Tighten your abdominal muscles. Exhale as you slowly stand up. Slowly sit down with control.

Reps: 8–12

Sets: 1–3

Tempo: 4–4

Rest: 30–90 seconds between sets

Tips and techniques:

- Press your heels against the floor and tighten your buttocks as you stand to help you balance.
- Steady yourself before you sit down.
- Exhale as you stand, inhale as you sit.

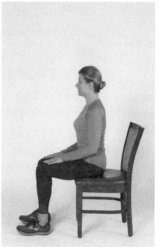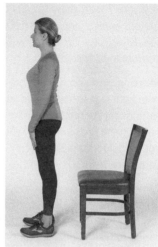

Make it easier: Rest, sitting on the chair, for a few seconds between reps when needed.

Make it harder: Cross your arms over your chest or place them behind your head. 🛡

Basic level: 10-Minute Cardio Interval Workout

Cardio exercise—also known as aerobic or endurance exercise—is any activity that gets you breathing a little harder and increases your heart rate for a sustained period. The intensity level can be low (such as walking your dog), moderate (brisk walking or Zumba), or high (running or kickboxing). This workout is high-intensity if you are moving vigorously, but it's low-impact, so it's easy on your joints. You'll get both cardio and strength benefits from this workout, along with improving coordination and balance—and it's fun!

It also qualifies as interval training, which repeatedly alternates short bursts of quick or vigorous exercise with bouts of easy activity to recover. This type of workout has been shown to deliver results in less time.

Instructions: As with any workout, you should begin with a warm-up. We recommend the warm-up routine on page 18. Don't forget to cool down afterward with an additional three to five minutes of easy marching in place, and then wrap up by doing the stretches on page 40 to improve your flexibility and range of motion.

To make sure you're doing this as an interval workout, do each exercise vigorously for 60 seconds, followed by 60 seconds of easy marching in place before moving on to the next exercise. If 60 seconds is too long for you to perform these exercises, you can do 30 seconds of each exercise and then repeat the entire series. You can shorten the recovery bout, too, or keep it at 60 seconds or even longer if you need more time to recover. If you want a longer workout, you can repeat the series as many times as you like.

Aim to do this workout two or three times a week, preferably on nonconsecutive days since it's a high-intensity workout.

What you need: Nothing.

1 | Charleston

The Charleston is a swing-style dance step that is fun to do, yet gets your heart rate up.

Starting position: Stand up straight with your feet together and your arms bent in front of you, palms facing away from your body.

Movement: Step forward with your left foot (1) and kick forward with your right leg (2). Place your right foot down just behind you (3) and then step back with your left foot and sink into a small lunge, front knee bent slightly, back leg straight (4). On each of these four counts, swing your arms from one side of your body to the other in an arc, with palms facing forward. Continue for 30 seconds. Repeat, stepping forward with the right foot and kicking with the left leg for 30 seconds.

When you've finished, march in place for 60 seconds before going on to the next exercise.

Tips and techniques:

• Keep your head up; don't look at your feet.

• Tighten your abdominal muscles.

• Don't collapse forward as you lunge back. Keep your chest lifted.

Make it easier: Take smaller steps. Kick lower. Step back without lunging. Make smaller arm movements.

Make it harder: Take bigger steps, kick higher, and lunge lower. Raise your arms above your head as you swing them.

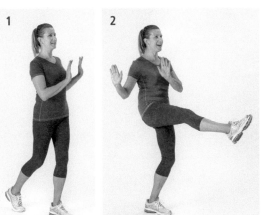
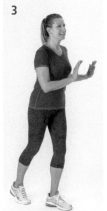
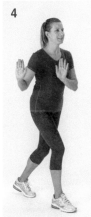

2 | Side lunge with knee lift

These work your body in the frontal plane (side-to-side motion), in contrast to more common forward motions (sagittal plane).

Starting position: Stand up straight with your feet together and your arms at your sides.

Movement: Step way out to the side with your left foot, while keeping your right foot in place. As your left foot hits the ground, transfer most of your weight to your left leg, hinge forward at your hips, and bend your left knee, lowering into a lunge. Keep your right leg straight and put your hands on your left thigh for support. Press into your left foot to stand back up, shifting your weight onto your right foot, and raise your left knee to hip level. Get your balance, and then step out with your left leg again for another lunge. Continue for 30 seconds. Repeat the sequence stepping out to the right for 30 seconds.

When you've finished, march in place for 60 seconds before going on to the next exercise.

Tips and techniques:

• Keep your spine neutral, your shoulders down and back, and your abdominal muscles tightened throughout.

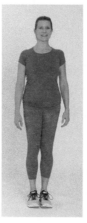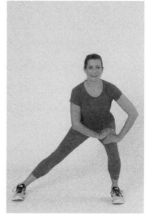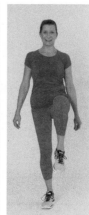

• Hinge at the hips as you lunge.
• Don't let the knee of the lunging leg extend beyond your toes.

Make it easier: Make the lunge smaller by not lowering so far down. Skip the knee lift.

Make it harder: Sit back farther into a lower lunge. Raise your arms overhead.

3 | Twist

Twists fire up your core muscles and provide movement in the transverse plane (rotational motion).

Starting position: Stand up straight with your feet together and your arms at your sides.

Movement: Bend your knees slightly, lift your heels off the floor, pivot on the balls of your feet, and rotate your lower body to the right, bringing your heels down, as you swing your arms to the left at chest height. Immediately rotate your lower body to the left as your arms go to the right. Continue alternating direction for 60 seconds.

When you've finished, march in place for 60 seconds before going on to the next exercise.

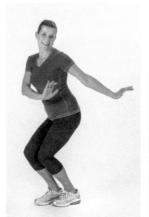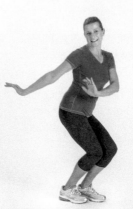

Tips and techniques:

• Keep the movement smooth, not jerky.
• Tighten your abdominal muscles.
• If you have low back problems, check with your doctor before doing this move.

Make it easier: Go slower. Don't bend your knees as much. Keep your arms low.

Make it harder: Bend your knees as you twist and see how low you can go. Raise your arms over your head as you twist.

4 | Modified burpee

A modified version of the classic burpee eliminates the jumps, providing total-body exercise that's more accessible to beginners and minimizes the impact on weight-bearing joints.

Starting position: Stand up straight with your feet together and your arms at your sides.

Movement: Squat down, placing your hands on the floor. Keeping your hands on the floor, step backward into a plank position. Bring your feet back in toward your hands. Then stand back up. Repeat for 60 seconds.

When you've finished, march in place for 60 seconds before going on to the next exercise.

Tips and techniques:

• Keep your head and neck in line with your spine.

• Keep your abdominal muscles tight.

Make it easier: Skip the plank portion. Simply squat down, touch the floor, and stand back up.

Make it harder: As you stand up, rise up onto the balls of your feet and reach overhead with your arms.

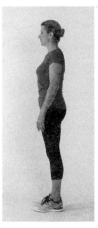 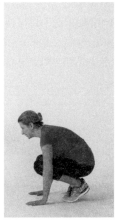 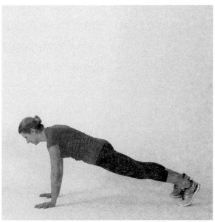 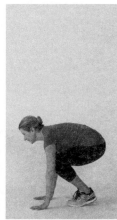 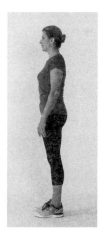

5 | Grapevine

This side-to-side step is a classic '80s aerobic dance move that improves coordination, even if you think you have two left feet.

Starting position: Stand up straight with your feet together and your arms at your sides.

Movement: Step with your left foot out to the side. Cross your right foot behind your left leg as you cross your forearms in front of you. Step with your left foot out to the side again, opening your arms out to the sides. Then bring your right foot next to your left one to return to the starting position. Repeat to the right, stepping with your right foot out to the side. Continue, alternating directions for 60 seconds.

When you've finished, march in place for 60 seconds.

Tips and techniques:

• Get comfortable with the footwork and then add the arms.

• Keep your shoulders and hips facing forward as you move from side to side.

• It's all right to look at your feet when you are learning the move, but after that, keep your head up.

Make it easier: Take smaller steps. Don't swing your arms out as high.

Make it harder: Take larger steps and add hops as you step. Reach overhead with your arms.

Note: *If you did intervals of 30 seconds instead of 60 seconds, repeat this entire series, to make a 10-minute workout.* ▼

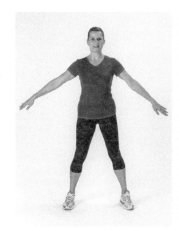 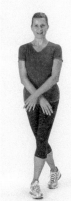 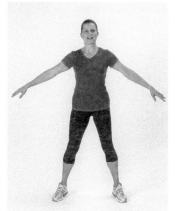 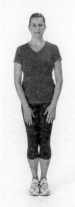

Challenge level: Strength Workout

This strength workout takes things up a notch, requiring not only greater strength but also better balance than the basic-level workout. It works all your major muscle groups for head-to-toe toning.

Instructions: If you're not already warmed up, begin by performing the warm-up routine on page 18. Cool down afterward with three to five minutes of easy marching in place, and then wrap up by doing the stretches on page 40.

Note that by speeding up your reps (see specific directions in the exercise descriptions), you can also turn this routine into a power training workout. To derive additional cardio benefits from this workout, do one set of each exercise with little to no rest between exercises, and then repeat the entire series one or two more times.

Aim to do this workout two or three times a week, preferably on nonconsecutive days.

What you need: Staircase or exercise stepper; exercise mat or thick towel or carpet; sturdy chair.

1 | Step-up

Step-ups help tone your gluteal and thigh muscles. If you're doing these on the bottom step of a staircase (as opposed to an exercise stepper), make sure you can grab the railing easily, if necessary.

Starting position: Stand facing a low step with your feet together. Relax your arms at your sides.

Movement: Place your right foot on the step. Slowly lift your body up onto the step, straightening your right leg. Hold. Keeping your weight on your right leg, slowly bend your right leg to lower yourself by a few inches, lightly touching the floor behind you with your left foot before rising back up for the next rep. Finish all reps with your right foot on the step, then repeat with your left foot on the step. This completes one set.

Reps: 8–12 on each side for strength, 6–10 on each side for power

Sets: 1–3

Tempo: 3–1–3 for strength, 1–1–3 for power

Rest: 30–90 seconds between sets

Tips and techniques:

- Stand up straight with your spine neutral and your shoulders down and back.
- Make sure your entire foot is on the step.
- Keep your abdominal muscles tight.

Make it easier: Use a lower step.

Make it harder: Use a higher step. Raise your arms overhead.

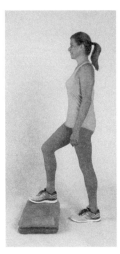 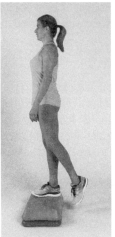 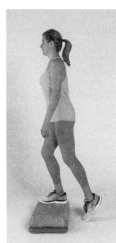

2 | Bench push-up

These are easier than traditional push-ups, because the semi-upright position reduces the amount of body weight you have to lift. The higher you place your hands, the easier the exercise will be.

Starting position: Place your hands shoulder-width apart on a bench (or desk, chair, or step). Walk your feet back so your body is at a 45° angle to the floor and forms a straight line from head to heels. Your heels should be off the floor.

Movement: Bend your elbows out to the sides and slowly lower your upper body toward the bench until your elbows are bent about 90°. Hold. Press against the bench and straighten your arms to return to the starting position.

Reps: 8–12 for strength, 6–10 for power

Sets: 1–3

Tempo: 3–1–3 for strength, 3–1–1 for power

Rest: 30–90 seconds between sets

Tips and techniques:

- Keep your head in line with your spine.
- Keep your abdominal muscles tight to prevent your back from arching too much.
- Don't bend at the hips.
- You can move your hands closer together or farther apart to work different muscles (see "Adjusting the challenge," page 16).

Make it easier: Use a higher bench or counter.

Make it harder: Use a lower bench or step, or do a full push-up on the floor.

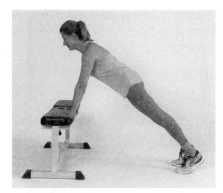
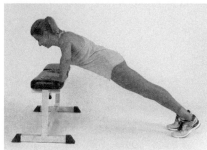

3 | Stationary lunge

These lunges will keep you strong and agile, so picking things up from the floor will be easier.

Starting position: Stand up straight with your right foot one to two feet in front of your left foot, hands on your hips. Shift your weight forward and lift your left heel off the floor.

Movement: Bend your knees and lower your torso straight down until your right thigh is about parallel to the floor. Hold, then return to the starting position. Finish all reps, then repeat with your left foot forward. This completes one set.

Reps: 8–12 on each side for strength, 6–10 on each side for power

Sets: 1–3

Tempo: 3–1–3 for strength, 3–1–1 for power

Rest: 30–90 seconds between sets

Tips and techniques:

- Keep your front knee directly over your ankle.
- In the lunge position, your shoulder, hip, and rear knee should be aligned. Don't lean forward or back.
- Keep your spine neutral and your shoulders down and back.

Make it easier: Lower your torso only halfway. Hold on to the back of a chair with one hand to help yourself balance.

Make it harder: Hold for four counts in the lunge position before returning to the starting position. Hold your arms overhead as you lunge.

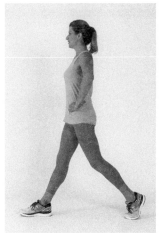
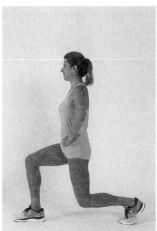

4 | Triceps dip

This classic exercise tones and strengthens the backsides of your upper arms. These muscles help when you're trying to open a stuck window.

Starting position: Place a bench or chair against a wall or on a mat so it doesn't move. Sit near the edge with your legs bent and feet flat on the floor. Place your hands next to your hips and grasp the edge. Pushing down on your hands, raise your buttocks and shift forward to clear the edge.

Movement: Bend your elbows back and lower your hips toward the floor. Keep your abdominal muscles tight. Hold, then straighten your arms to return to the starting position.

Reps: 8–12 for strength, 6–10 for power

Sets: 1–3

Tempo: 3–1–3 for strength, 3–1–1 for power

Rest: 30–90 seconds between sets

Tips and techniques:

• Keep your shoulders down and back, away from your ears.

• Bend your elbows no farther than 90°.

• Keep your back close to the bench or chair.

Make it easier: Lower yourself a shorter distance.

Make it harder: Do one-leg dips by crossing one leg over the other. Or, extend your legs straight out in front of you so you're balancing on your heels.

If you have any shoulder issues, check with your doctor before doing this exercise.

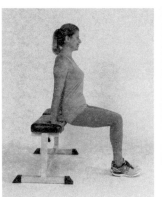 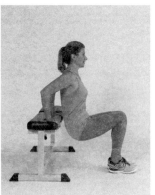 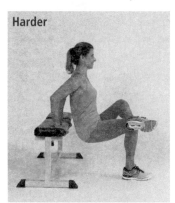

Harder

5 | Wall squat

These squats may look easy, but they can provide a killer thigh workout if you hold the position longer.

Starting position: Stand up straight and place your back against a wall. Walk your feet out about 18 to 24 inches. Place your hands on your hips.

Movement: Slowly bend your knees and hips, sliding your back down the wall. Stop before your buttocks reach knee level. Hold. Slowly straighten your legs as you return to the starting position.

Reps: 8–12 for strength, 6–10 for power

Sets: 1–3

Tempo: 4–2–4 for strength, 4–2–1 for power

Rest: 30–90 seconds between sets

Tips and techniques:

• Maintain a neutral spine, with your shoulders down and back.

• Your knees should be aligned over your ankles in the squat position. Adjust your foot position, if necessary, to maintain proper alignment.

• Keep your knees pointing forward. Don't let them roll in or out as you squat.

Make it easier: Slide down a shorter distance, doing a smaller squat.

Make it harder: Hold each squat for four counts.

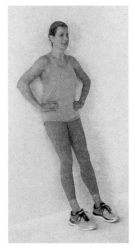 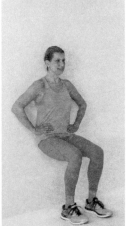

6 | Superman

Channel your inner superhero, while strengthening the back muscles that help you stand tall.

Starting position: Lie facedown on the floor with your legs together and your arms extended, palms down.

Movement: Simultaneously lift your arms, head, chest, and legs up off the floor as high as is comfortable. Hold. Return to the starting position.

Reps: 8–12 for strength, 6–10 for power

Sets: 1–3

Tempo: 4–2–4 for strength, 1–2–4 for power

Rest: 30–90 seconds between sets

Tips and techniques:

• Tighten your buttocks before lifting.

• Don't look up.

• Keep your shoulders down, away from your ears.

Make it easier: Lift only your arms, and then lift only your legs, to make one rep.

Make it harder: Hold for four counts before lowering.

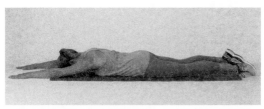
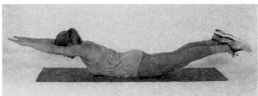

7 | Plank with leg lift

Full planks are tough enough, but adding a leg lift increases the challenge.

Starting position: Kneel on all fours with your hands and knees directly aligned under your shoulders and hips.

Movement: Tighten your abdominal muscles, walk your hands out in front of you, and lower your upper body onto your forearms. Align your shoulders directly over your elbows. Raise your knees off the floor, extend your legs, and lift one foot off the floor, so you are balancing on your forearms and the toes and ball of one foot. Your body should be in line from head to heels. Hold. If you held for less than 30 seconds, repeat. For example, if you can hold a plank for 15 seconds, you would do two reps. Then repeat, lifting the other leg.

Reps: as many as needed to hold for a total of 30 seconds on each leg

Sets: 1

Hold: up to 30 seconds on each leg

Rest: 30–90 seconds between reps

Tips and techniques:

• Keep your neck and spine neutral during the plank.

• Tighten your abdominal muscles so your belly doesn't sag toward the floor.

• Keep your shoulders down and back.

• Look at the floor in front of you. Don't look up.

Make it easier: Place your knees on the floor.

Make it harder: Work up to holding each leg up for 60 seconds. You can rest in between. ◗

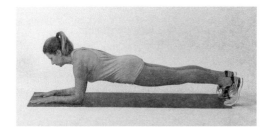
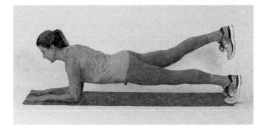

    Body-Weight Exercise

Challenge level: Core Workout

The muscles in your abdomen, back, sides, pelvis, hips, and buttocks make up your core, which is responsible for coordinating movement between your upper and lower body and maintaining good posture. This workout adds more balance challenges to engage your core and improve your balance, stability, posture, and power.

Instructions: If you're not already warmed up, begin by performing the warm-up routine on page 18 to prepare your body for more vigorous activity. Finish by doing the stretches on page 40 to improve your flexibility and range of motion.

Aim to do this workout two or three times a week, preferably on nonconsecutive days.

What you need: Exercise mat or thick towel or carpet.

1 | Squat with knee lift and rotation

These get you moving in all three planes of motion for a trio of benefits: strength, coordination, and balance.

Starting position: Stand up straight with your feet together and your arms at your sides.

Movement: Step out to the right, hinge at your hips, and bend your knees to lower your buttocks into a squat as if sitting in a chair. At the same time, clasp your hands loosely in front of your chest. As you stand back up, raise your right knee and rotate your upper body to the right. Return to the squat for the next rep. Finish all reps, then repeat the sequence stepping out to the left. This completes one set.

Reps: 8–12 on each side

Sets: 1–3

Tempo: 3–3

Rest: 30–90 seconds between sets

Tips and techniques:

- Keep your spine neutral and your shoulders down and back.
- Don't let your knees extend beyond your toes; if you look down you should be able to see your toes.
- As you hinge your upper body slightly forward, keep your chest lifted.

Make it easier: As you stand up, lift one knee up in front of you without twisting. If this is still too challenging, simply do squats without a knee lift or rotation.

Make it harder: Hold the squat, the knee lift, or both for two to four counts.

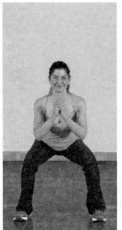 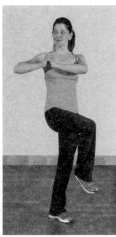

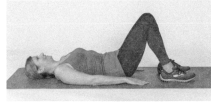
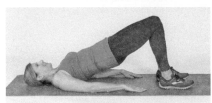
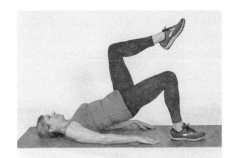

2 | Bridge with knee lift

Adding a balance challenge to this staple exercise really fires up your core muscles.

Starting position: Lie on your back with your knees bent and feet flat on the floor, hip-width apart. Place your arms at your sides. Relax your shoulders against the floor.

Movement: Tighten your buttocks, then lift your hips up off the floor as high as is comfortable. Keep your hips even and spine neutral. Pull your left knee in toward your chest, keeping your pelvis level. Hold. Lower your left foot. Pull your right knee in toward your chest. Hold. Lower your right foot, and then slowly lower your buttocks to the floor.

Reps: 8–12

Sets: 1–3

Tempo: 3–2–1–2–2–1–2–3

Rest: 30–90 seconds between sets

Tips and techniques:
- Tighten your buttocks before lifting.
- Keep your shoulders, hips, knees, and feet evenly aligned.
- Keep your shoulders down and relaxed against the floor.

Make it easier: Lower to the floor between knee lifts. Or do bridges without knee lifts.

Make it harder: Hold each knee lift for a count of two to four.

3 | Diagonal opposite arm and leg raise

The arm and leg movements add motion in multiple planes, so your core muscles have to work harder.

Starting position: Kneel on all fours with your hands and knees directly aligned under your shoulders and hips. Keep your head and spine neutral.

Movement: Extend your left leg off the floor behind you while reaching out in front of you with your right arm. Keeping your hips and shoulders squared, try to bring that leg and arm parallel to the floor. Hold. Move your extended arm and leg outward on a diagonal. Think of a clock: instead of noon and 6, move them to 1 and 7. Hold. Return your arm and leg to the center and then back to the starting position. Repeat with your right leg and left arm (pointing to 11 and 5 on the imaginary clock). This is one rep.

Reps: 8–12

Sets: 1–3

Tempo: 3–1–2–1–5

Rest: 30–90 seconds between sets

Tips and techniques:
- Keep your shoulders and hips squared to maintain alignment throughout.
- Keep your neck and spine neutral.
- Think of pulling your hand and leg in opposite directions, lengthening your torso.

Make it easier: Don't move your arm and leg on a diagonal; just lift and lower.

Make it harder: Hold the raised and diagonal positions for two to four counts.

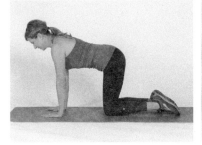
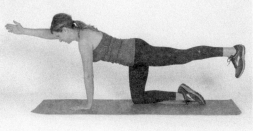
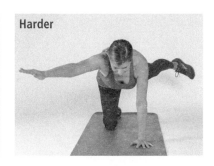

Harder

4 | Plank with knee drop

This exercise turns a stationary core toner into an active exercise to challenge muscles in a different way and keep you on your toes.

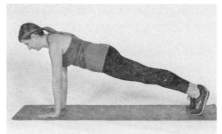 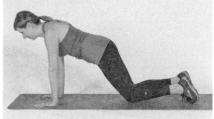

Starting position: Kneel on all fours with your hands and knees directly aligned under your shoulders and hips. Extend both legs with your feet flexed and toes touching the floor so that you are balancing on your palms, toes, and balls of your feet, like the top position of a push-up. This is the plank.

Movement: Tighten your abdominal muscles. Lower both knees toward the floor, then extend your legs again to return to the plank position.

Reps: 8–12

Sets: 1–3

Tempo: 3–3

Rest: 30–90 seconds between sets

Tips and techniques:

- Keep your neck and spine neutral during the plank.

- Keep your shoulders down and back.
- Breathe comfortably.

Make it easier: Do fewer reps and gradually work up to eight to 12. Or skip the knee drops and simply hold the plank.

Make it harder: Hold the knee drop position for one to four counts.

5 | Clam

Clams are a key rehab exercise, but too much sitting has made them necessary for almost everyone to stabilize the pelvis and avoid injuries.

Starting position: Lie on your right side, knees bent and heels in line with your buttocks. Rest your head on your right arm and place your left hand on the floor in front of you.

Movement: Engage your gluteal muscles and lift your left knee up toward the ceiling, keeping your feet together. Hold. Then slowly lower to the starting position. Finish all reps, then repeat on the other side. This completes one set.

Reps: 8–12 on each side

Sets: 1–3

Tempo: 3–1–3

Rest: 30–90 seconds between sets

Tips and techniques:

- Keep your hips stacked and still throughout the movement.

- You don't have to lift high. Think about rotating your thighbone while keeping your pelvis stable. If you feel the effort in your buttock, you're doing it correctly.

- Don't roll forward or back as you lift. 🛡

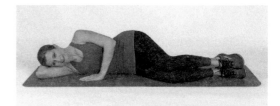

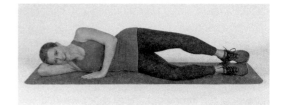

Challenge level: 10-Minute Cardio Interval Workout

This combo cardio and strength workout will kick your metabolism into high gear thanks to speedy, jumping moves (plyometrics) that rev up your heart rate and help to strengthen your bones along with your muscles. Unlike the basic-level 10-Minute Cardio Interval Workout (page 27), which is low-impact, this one consists of jumping exercises, which are by definition high-impact. Before starting, be sure to read the jumping safety tips on page 14.

You'll find five high-intensity, high-impact exercises in this workout. But you won't go directly from one to the next. Instead, we've planned this as an interval workout, in which you repeatedly alternate vigorous exercise with more moderate activity to recover. High-intensity interval workouts amp up your benefits in less time, and they can keep your metabolism revved up for a longer period of time post-exercise than more moderate levels of activity.

Instructions: Start with the warm-up routine on page 18 to prepare your body for more vigorous activity. Remember to cool down afterward with an additional three to five minutes of easy marching in place, and then wrap up by doing the stretches on page 40 to improve your flexibility and range of motion.

To make sure you're doing this as an interval workout, do each exercise for 60 seconds, followed by 60 seconds of easy marching in place to bring down the intensity level and catch your breath. If 60 seconds of each exercise feels like too much, you can do 30 seconds of each one and then repeat the entire series. You can shorten the recovery bout to 30 seconds, too, or keep it at 60 seconds or even longer if you need more time to recover.

Aim to do this workout two or three times a week, preferably on nonconsecutive days.

What you need: Nothing.

1 | Knee hop

This move is reminiscent of skipping, so channel your inner child for this one. If you have space to move forward, feel free to do so.

Starting position: Stand up straight with your feet together.

Movement: Raise your left knee up to about hip height, hopping a little bit off the floor with your right foot as you lift. Immediately repeat on your other leg. Continue alternating legs. Let your arms swing naturally.

When you've finished, march in place for 60 seconds before going on to the next exercise.

Tips and techniques:

• Keep your head up.

• Don't hunch or round your shoulders forward.

• Keep your abdominal muscles tight.

Make it easier: Don't lift your knees as high. Don't hop as high.

Make it harder: Lift your knee higher. Hop higher or faster.

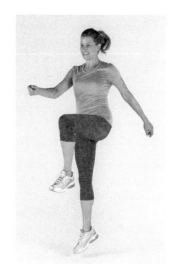

2 | Side hop

This exercise mixes things up by training your body laterally—a direction you probably don't move in often.

Starting position: Stand up straight with your feet together.

Movement: Shift your weight onto your right foot and leap to your left, landing with your left foot, followed by your right one. Repeat, hopping to your right. You can hold your arms in front of you or let them swing naturally.

When you've finished, march in place for 60 seconds before going on to the next exercise.

Tips and techniques:

- Don't hunch or round your shoulders forward.
- Keep your abdominal muscles tight.

Make it easier: Hop a shorter distance to the side and stay lower to the floor.

Make it harder: Make your hops bigger and higher.

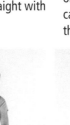
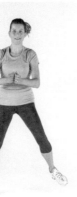
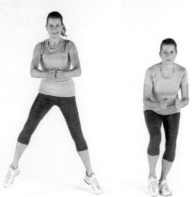

3 | Diagonal knee pull with hop

This works the oblique muscles, which wrap around your torso and enable you to twist and bend sideways.

Starting position: Stand up straight with your feet shoulder-width apart and your arms overhead and angled to the right.

Movement: Hop as you raise your left knee across your body. At the same time, pull your arms down toward your knee and across your body. Lower your knee and extend your arms back to the starting position, but just lightly touch your foot to the floor before hopping into another knee pull. Repeat for 30 seconds with your left leg, and then switch legs and repeat for another 30 seconds.

When you've finished, march in place for 60 seconds before going on to the next exercise.

Tips and techniques:

- Keep your head up.
- Tighten your abdominal muscles.
- Keep your torso straight as you bring your hands down and knee up.
- Keep your shoulders down and back, away from your ears.

Make it easier: Skip the arm movements and just do the knee lifts at a slower pace. You can put your hands on your hips if that's more comfortable.

Make it harder: Go faster, lift your knee higher, and really pull your arms down. Also, contract your abdominal muscles with each pull-down as if you are doing crunches.

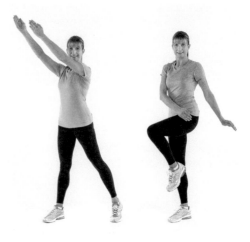

4 | Jumping jacks

Jumping jacks may be old-school, but they really get your heart rate up.

Starting position: Stand up straight with your feet together and your arms at your sides.

Movement: Jump, spreading your feet apart beyond shoulder-width, as you raise your arms out to the sides and up over your head. Jump again, bringing your feet back together while moving your arms out to the sides and down.

When you've finished, march in place for 60 seconds before going on to the next exercise.

Tips and techniques:

- Don't hunch or round your shoulders forward.
- Keep your abdominal muscles tight.
- Keep your shoulders down and back, away from your ears.

Make it easier: Don't spread your feet as far apart when you jump; stay lower to the floor.

Make it harder: Make your jumps higher and faster.

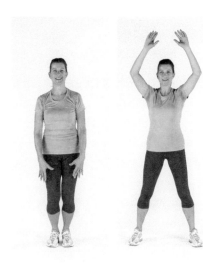

5 | Burpee

Burpees provide serious exercise, working the entire body and quickly cranking up your heart rate and calorie burn.

Starting position: Stand up straight with your feet together and your arms at your sides.

Movement: Squat down, placing your hands on the floor. Jump your legs back behind you into plank position. Jump your feet back in toward your hands. Jump up into the air, raising your arms overhead, and land in the starting position.

When you've finished, march in place for 60 seconds.

Tips and techniques:

- Keep your head and neck in line with your spine.
- Keep your abdominal muscles tight.

Make it easier: Step your feet in and out of the plank position instead of jumping. Make the jump lower.

Make it harder: Make your jump higher. Move more quickly from one position to the next.

Note: If you did intervals of 30 seconds instead of 60 seconds, repeat this entire series, to make a 10-minute work-out.

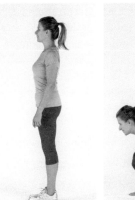 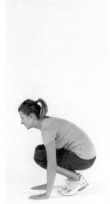 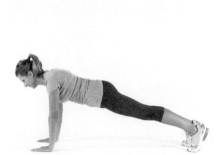 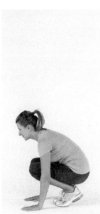 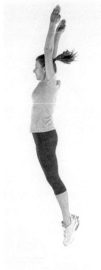

Post-workout stretches

The hard part of your workout is over, but before you call it a day, it's important to spend a few minutes stretching. As tempting as it may be to skip stretching and get on with the rest of your day, it's worth the effort. As you get older, muscles and joints get stiffer, making it harder to do things like reaching overhead or washing your back. The end of your workout is the perfect time to stretch because your muscles are more pliable and your joints are looser from the previous activity. This allows you to stretch a little farther to maintain, or even increase, flexibility and range of motion.

Instructions: For optimal results, hold each stretch for 10 to 30 seconds, and repeat it one to five times for a total of 60 seconds.

Safety tips: When stretching, please remember:
- Breathe normally.
- Don't bounce.
- Don't overextend your body. Stretch only to the point of mild tension, never pain. If a stretch hurts, stop immediately.

For additional measures, see "Stretching safety tips," page 14.

If you have had a joint replaced or repaired, ask your surgeon whether you need to avoid certain stretches, such as the torso rotation. If you have osteoporosis, consult your doctor before doing floor stretches or stretches that bend the spine.

What you need: Exercise mat or thick towel or carpet; sturdy chair.

1 | Calf stretch

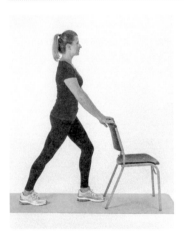

This stretches the gastrocnemius (the largest calf muscle) which is activated when you push off with your back foot while walking; it helps prevent certain foot problems.

Starting position: Hold the back of a chair or press your hands against a wall, arms extended at shoulder height.

Movement: Extend your right leg straight back and press the heel into the floor. Allow your left knee to bend, keeping both heels grounded on the floor. Feel the stretch up your right calf. Hold. Return to the starting position. Finish all reps, then repeat with your left leg back.

Reps: 2–6 on each side

Hold: 10–30 seconds

Tips and techniques:
- Hold a full-body lean from the ankle as you stretch.
- Step closer to the chair or wall if you find yourself bending at the waist and leaning forward.
- Keep your front knee over your ankle.

2 | Soleus stretch

This targets the deep muscle in your calves, which aids in balance by preventing you from falling forward.

Starting position: Hold the back of a chair or press your hands against a wall, arms extended at shoulder height.

Movement: Extend your right leg behind you about half of the distance as for the calf stretch (at left) and press the heel into the floor. Allow your left knee to bend as you do so, while keeping the heel grounded on the floor. Now bend your right knee as much as possible, pressing into your right heel until you feel a stretch low in your calf. Hold. Return to the starting position. Finish all reps, then repeat with your left leg back.

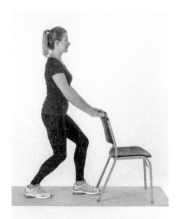

Reps: 2–6 on each side

Hold: 10–30 seconds

Tips and techniques:
- Don't bend at your waist.
- Keep your front knee directly over your ankle.
- Step closer to the chair or wall if you are having trouble maintaining good form.

3 | Quad stretch

This move focuses on the muscles in the front of your thighs, which are key walking muscles but get tight from too much sitting.

Starting position: Stand up straight, feet together, holding the back of a chair with both hands.

Movement: Bend your right knee and reach back with your right hand to grasp your foot, lifting it toward your right buttock. Feel the stretch in the front of your thigh. Hold. Slowly lower your foot to the floor. Finish all reps, then repeat with your other leg.

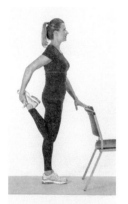

Reps: 2–6 on each side

Hold: 10–30 seconds

Tips and techniques:

- Try to keep both knees together, with the bent knee pointing toward the floor.
- Keep your pelvis neutral; don't arch your back.
- If you have trouble grasping your foot, place a strap or belt around it to assist with the stretch.

4 | Hamstring stretch

This stretch will improve your flexibility when you bend from the waist and will help you to touch your toes or pick things up from the floor.

Starting position: Stand up straight with your arms at your sides.

Movement: Extend your left leg straight in front of you, heel grounded on the floor and toes pointing to the ceiling. Place your hands on your right thigh for support and hinge forward from the hip, keeping your spine neutral. Bend your right knee until you feel a stretch up the back of your left thigh. Hold. Return to the starting position. Finish all reps, then repeat with your right leg forward.

Reps: 2–6 on each side

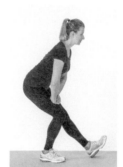

Hold: 10–30 seconds

Tips and techniques:

- As you hinge forward, keep your chest lifted and imagine your chin reaching toward your foot.
- Keep your shoulders down and back, away from your ears.
- Ease off the stretch if you feel any pressure behind the knee or in your back.

5 | Chest and shoulder stretch

This move helps counteract the hunching done while using cellphones, tablets, and computers.

Starting position: Stand up straight with your arms at your sides.

Movement: Bring your hands behind your back and lace your fingers, palms facing up. Roll your shoulders back and down. Then, gently lift your hands up and away from you as far as comfortably possible. Hold. Return to the starting position.

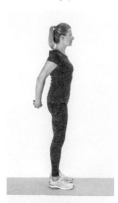

Reps: 2–6

Hold: 10–30 seconds

Tips and techniques:

- Keep your shoulders down and back, away from your ears, as you stretch.
- Look straight ahead, keeping your chin level with the floor.
- Don't lean forward or arch your back.

6 | Hip flexor stretch

This stretch helps prevent the low back pain that can occur when the muscles at the tops of your thighs are too tight.

Starting position: Kneel with your hands at your sides.

Movement: Put your left leg in front of you with the knee bent at a 90° angle and foot flat on the floor. Place your hands on your left thigh for support. Shift your weight forward, pressing into the front of the hip of your right leg while keeping the top of your right foot on the floor. Feel the stretch in the front of your right thigh and hip. Hold. Return to the starting position. Finish all reps, then repeat with your right leg forward.

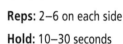

Reps: 2–6 on each side

Hold: 10–30 seconds

Tips and techniques:

- Keep your front knee over your ankle, not jutting out past your toes.
- Keep your head and spine neutral, your shoulders down and back, and your abdominal muscles tightened.
- Keep your pelvis neutral, not tucked under or lifted.

7 | Torso twist

This stretch helps maintain your ability to rotate and look over your shoulder, as you need to do when driving.

Starting position: Sit up straight on the floor with your legs extended in front of you. Bend your right leg and place your right foot on the floor by the outside of your left knee.

Movement: Slowly rotate your head and torso to the right side, placing your right hand on the floor behind you for support and your left hand on the outside of your right knee to help you stretch farther. Feel the stretch in your back and neck. Hold. Slowly return to the starting position. Finish all reps, then repeat in the other direction.

Reps: 2–6 to each side

Hold: 10–30 seconds

Tips and techniques:

• Flex the foot of your extended leg.

• Use the hand on the floor behind you to help you sit up straight.

• Each time you rotate, choose a spot to focus on while holding. This spot should move noticeably as your range of motion improves.

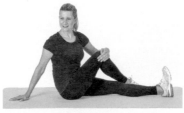

8 | Pretzel stretch

This stretch targets the muscles in the outer thigh and hip, which can lead to knee problems when tight.

Starting position: Lie on your back with your left knee bent and your foot flat on the floor. Rest your right ankle on your left thigh, just above your left knee. Your right knee should point out to the side. Grasp the back of your left thigh with both hands.

Movement: Slowly draw your left leg toward you, lifting your left foot off the floor, until you feel the stretch in your right hip and buttock. Hold. Return to the starting position. Finish all reps, then repeat with your left ankle on your right thigh.

Reps: 2–6 on each side

Hold: 10–30 seconds

Tips and techniques:

• Keep your shoulders down and back, relaxing them against the floor.

• Keep your head on the floor and your neck relaxed.

• If it's too hard to grasp your thigh with both hands, put a strap or small towel around the back of the thigh and hold both ends.

9 | Child pose three ways

This variation on the classic child pose improves flexibility in your back, arms, shoulders, and sides.

Starting position: Kneel on all fours, knees apart, big toes touching, and head and neck in line with your spine.

Movement: This is a three-part stretch. Slowly drop your buttocks back toward your heels as you extend your hands in front of you and rest your forehead on the mat. Feel the stretch down your arms, shoulders, and back. Hold. Then walk your hands diagonally out to the right and place your left hand on top of your right hand. Feel the stretch down the left side of your body and your back. Hold. Then walk your hands diagonally out to the left and place your right hand

on top of your left hand. Feel the stretch down the right side of your body and your back. Hold. Return to the starting position.

Reps: 2–6 on each side

Hold: 10–30 seconds

Tips and techniques:

• You can adjust how far apart your knees are so that you are comfortable.

• Lower your buttocks only as far as feels comfortable. If necessary, place a pillow or towel between your thighs and calves to limit the stretch.

• Keep your shoulders down and back, away from your ears. ♦

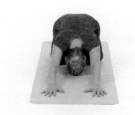
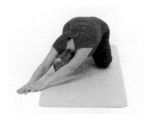
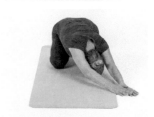

Staying motivated

Exercise is easy when you're excited about trying a new workout or seeing quick results. The challenge is sticking with it over the long haul. But that's when the benefits really start to stack up. A short-term exercise program might help you tone up your muscles in advance of a beach vacation or a high school reunion. But only a long-term program will get you looking and feeling better for years to come. Consistency is key.

For example, a study published in the American Heart Association's journal *Circulation* found that a regular exercise program helped sedentary middle-aged men and women reverse the damage to their circulatory systems from too much couch time. Their VO2 max (a measure of aerobic capacity) increased by 18% at a time of life when it's usually declining, and the stiffness of the heart's left ventricle decreased by 29%, reducing the risk that these men and women would suffer heart failure in old age. But it required work. These measurements were taken at the end of two years, during which the participants had been exercising four or five days every week.

Can the promise of far-off benefits sustain you when you're juggling a dozen responsibilities that need your attention right now? If you're like many people, the answer is no. Fortunately, there are strategies you can adopt to keep exercise from slipping lower on your to-do list—and help you develop a lifelong fitness habit. This chapter explores some of these tried-and-true approaches.

Find the motivation

Motivation can come from many sources. Since the most successful strategy varies from one individual to another, you may have to try multiple approaches to find what works best for you. Here are some suggestions to get you going—and keep you moving well into the future.

Change your mindset. Your mind is a powerful tool that can make or break your success. Try to think of yourself as an active person, someone who exercises regularly and enjoys movement. Creating a new identity that aligns with the goals you're trying to achieve is key to making healthy lifestyle changes like exercising regularly, according to *Atomic Habits* by James Clear. When you start to believe new things about yourself, like "I'm an exerciser," "I'm an active person," or "I feel better when I move," then taking the actions of an exerciser—like making time to work out, planning active get-togethers with friends, or trying a new activity like stand-up paddleboarding—will be easier.

Appreciate the joy of movement. Throughout this report, we've been sharing with you all of the complexity, ability, and beauty of the human body. Now, it's your turn to pay attention to just how

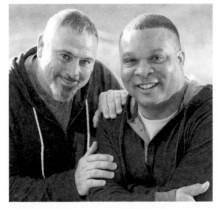

Invite a friend to work out with you. A workout buddy can help you stick to your exercise program. If you can't meet in person, do a session at home via FaceTime.

remarkable every movement that you make really is. Revel in the joy of being able to move your body in so many ways. If you take your body for granted and don't regularly exercise it, your mobility will become limited over time. So take care of it now.

Make it personal. There are many reasons to exercise, starting with fitness and health. But is there a more personal goal that can help keep you on track? Not for your doctor so he or she stops bugging you about your high blood pressure. Not for your spouse. Not for your kids. Not for some cultural ideal of how you should look. But for *you*. Maybe you want to get down on the floor and play with your grandkids. Maybe you want to take that walking tour in Italy after retirement. For one client, it was her passion for birding that spurred her on. By staying fit, she was able to hike to remote areas to see exotic birds. What activities would fitness make possible or more enjoyable for you, so you could keep doing it for years to come? Hiking? Golfing? Traveling? Find your passion or purpose and use it to fuel your workouts. Then, when you feel like quitting, think about why you started.

Harness positive memories. Some people struggle to find a type of exercise they enjoy. For them, machines at the gym may not cut it. A common strategy for helping to find exercise that you enjoy is to think about what you liked doing as a kid. It turns out that reminisc-

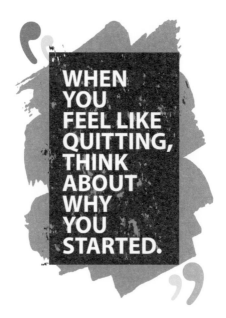

WHEN YOU FEEL LIKE QUITTING, THINK ABOUT WHY YOU STARTED.

ing may also inspire you to exercise more. When college students were prompted to recall a positive memory that would motivate them to exercise, they worked out more the following week than those who didn't try this approach, according to a study in the journal *Memory*. Even negative memories motivated some people to increase their exercise, because they served as a reminder of the need to improve. However, they were not as powerful as positive memories.

Switch up your workouts. Doing the same workouts over and over can become boring, and you may also find that your gains level off over time, if you're doing the same exercises repeatedly. Switching up your workouts can keep you on your toes by offering new challenges. At the end of this report, we've included two bonus workouts. Harvard Health Publishing also offers a range of exercise reports that provide more options,

whether your interest is yoga, tai chi, running, walking, or other cardio or strength workouts (see "Resources," page 52).

Make your intentions public. Telling others about your goals can help you stay on track because you know they'll ask you how you're doing. In fact, when you share your intentions with friends and family members, ask them to help you succeed by checking in with you regularly about your progress. You can also do this by sharing your workouts on Facebook or other social media. Words of encouragement from others can be very motivating.

Get a workout buddy. Invite a friend or relative to start exercising with you. Doing it together—even via FaceTime or Zoom if you can't meet in person—will keep you both accountable and make it more fun. Knowing that you are checking in with each other periodically will encourage you to stick to your routine.

Add music. Music makes workouts more fun, so you'll be more likely to do them in the first place. It can also inspire you once you start moving. Exercisers who listen to music tend to go longer and harder. Any upbeat tunes can add energy to your reps and keep you motivated.

Plan simple rewards. Give yourself a pat on the back for every step toward success, whether large or small. Blast your favorite tune during your cool-down. Text a friend after a workout so he or she can cheer you on. Treat yourself to a relaxing bath before bed with a beautifully scented bath oil. A bigger reward for staying on track toward your goal for a month might be new workout clothes or a massage.

Make a detailed plan

A goal without a plan is just a wish, as some witty sage once said. In fact, multiple studies support the idea that creating a plan for being more physically active will increase your likelihood of being successful. To help you sketch out a program, go to "My action plan," page 46.

Be kind to yourself

Don't beat yourself up if you miss a workout, or even an entire week. It's going to happen. Instead of the drill sergeant approach, try a little self-compassion. Treat yourself the way you'd treat a friend when he or she is struggling. Be supportive. Help problem-solve. Recognize all the progress you've made so far.

Behavior change researchers are finding that lack of self-compassion may be a key obstacle to making healthy lifestyle changes. While berating yourself sets up a negative spiral of self-criticism (which is more likely to lead to less healthy behaviors, like plopping on the couch with a carton of ice cream), research shows that being kind to yourself can stop that downward spiral and help you to learn from your experience, so you'll do better in the future. Here are some ways you can give yourself a break.

Be more flexible. No, this isn't about touching your toes. It's about being flexible about your workouts. You'll be more successful and feel better about yourself if you give up the perfectionist ideals that you have to work out for at least 30 minutes, you've got to go to the gym or take a class, or even that you've got to break a sweat. There are many, many ways to get a workout, and even one or two minutes at a time counts. In a study by University of Michigan behavior change scientist Michelle Segar, author of *No Sweat: How the Simple Science of Motivation Can Bring You a Lifetime of Fitness*, women who gave themselves permission to do what they could and feel good about it were happier and more active. Next time your exercise plans don't go as expected, adopt this it's-not-the-end-of-the-world attitude and see if you find it easier to get back on track.

Watch your language. Banish the words "should," "have to," and "can't" from your vocabulary when planning your exercise program. The language you use affects both how you feel and how you view exercise. Instead of negative statements, practice positive ones, such as "I can do this!" "Look how well I did yesterday (or last week)!" and "I am getting stronger." These verbal reinforcements will help exercise feel less like a chore and more like a privilege—something you "get to do" rather than something you "have to do." Any time you

notice toxic thoughts or negative language creep in, think—or say aloud—"Stop!"

Let exercise be its own reward

One of the many benefits of exercise is that it's not only good for you, it also feels good. Once you form an exercise habit, your daily workout will become something you don't want to miss, because you just feel better when you do it. Exercise eases pent-up anxiety and lifts your mood as endorphins (naturally occurring chemicals that make you feel good) flood your system. You feel better physically, too. Increased circulation brings more oxygen to your muscles and your brain, giving you energy. You grow stronger. Stiff joints loosen up. You sleep better at night.

You may also find that exercise helps you look better, as you tone your muscles. And if creeping weight gain has been an issue for you, exercise can help keep it in check.

In these multifaceted ways, exercise eventually becomes its own motivation. The trick is to keep doing it long enough to make a habit of it. One study found that it took an average of 66 days for a new behavior to become automatic—that is, a habit. Missing once or twice didn't derail people, but frequent inconsistency did. So keep nudging yourself in the right direction. You may be surprised to find yourself eager to get moving every day. ♥

My action plan

Start by answering these questions; then use that information to fill out your weekly log. Once the workouts are on your calendar, treat them like important appointments you can't miss. To make sure you don't backslide, think about the obstacles that might interfere with meeting your goal, and brainstorm ways to overcome these obstacles.

▶ What three workouts will you do this week? Choose one cardio, one strength, and one core workout.

Cardio (2 or 3 times per week): _____

Strength (2 or 3 times per week): _____

Core (3 to 5 times per week): _____

	SUNDAY	MONDAY	TUESDAY	WEDNESDAY	
What will you do?					
When will you do it?					
Where will you do it?					
With whom will you do it?					
How long will you do it?					

▶ When will you do the workouts? _____

▶ Where will you do the workouts? (This is usually an easy one when you're doing body-weight exercises.) _____

▶ With whom will you work out? (It's okay to go solo, too.) _____ _____

▶ How long will you work out? _____

THURSDAY	FRIDAY	SATURDAY

What are three barriers that could interfere with your workouts?

1. _____

2. _____

3. _____

What are three ways that you could overcome each of these obstacles?

Barrier #1

1. _____
_____

2. _____
_____

3. _____
_____

Barrier #2

1. _____
_____

2. _____
_____

3. _____
_____

Barrier #3

1. _____
_____

2. _____
_____

3. _____
_____

Bonus: Balance Workout

Balance training isn't just for older adults at risk of falling. Nearly everything you do—from getting out of bed and walking up and down stairs to getting in and out of your car and going out dancing—requires some degree of balance. When you start to do body-weight exercises, you may discover that your balance isn't as good as you thought it was. That's because body-weight exercises require more coordination and balance than you need when using exercise machines. If you've noticed any wobbling or feel unstable as you do the main workouts, adding this workout to your routine can help.

These exercises can ward off further decline, protect you from injury, make everyday tasks easier, improve athletic performance, and ensure that you can properly and safely execute the other body-weight exercises in this report. They also build some strength, especially in your lower body and core.

Instructions: Aim to do balance workouts two or three times a week. You can do them daily, if you like. If needed, you can hold on to the back of a chair or counter for support, or stand in the corner of a room so you can touch the walls to steady yourself. To help you execute the moves, engage your core muscles before you start each exercise, and pick a spot or object in front of you to focus on.

What you need: Sturdy chair (optional), counter (optional).

1 | Tandem standing

Even though you're stationary, this exercise requires your muscles to make microadjustments to keep you upright.

Starting position: Stand up straight, feet hip-width apart and weight evenly distributed on both feet. Put your arms at your sides and brace your abdominal muscles.

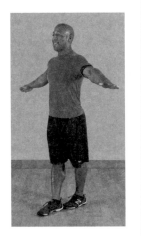

Movement: Place your right foot directly in front of your left foot, heel to toe, and squeeze your inner thighs together. Lift your arms out to your sides at shoulder level to help you balance. Hold. Return to the starting position, then repeat with your left foot in front. This is one rep.

Reps: 10

Sets: 1–3

Tempo: 2–2–2

Tips and techniques:
- Tighten your abdominal muscles, buttocks, and inner thighs to assist with balance.
- Keep your shoulders down and back.

Make it easier: Separate the feet a few inches.

Make it harder: Hold the position for 60 seconds; close your eyes.

2 | Single-leg stance

Balancing on one leg without moving is harder than it sounds and reminds you to keep your core muscles engaged for better stability.

Starting position: Stand up straight, feet together and weight evenly distributed on both feet. Relax your arms at your sides.

Movement: Bend your right knee enough to raise your right foot a few inches off the floor, and balance on your left leg. Hold. Lower your foot to the starting position, then repeat, balancing on your right leg.

Reps: 1

Sets: 1–3

Hold: 5–30 seconds

Tips and techniques:
- Maintain good posture throughout by keeping your chest lifted, your shoulders down and back, and your abdominal muscles braced.
- Extend your arms out to the sides if you are wobbly.

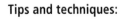

Make it easier: Keep the toes of your raised leg lightly touching the floor.

Make it harder: Hold for 60 seconds; close your eyes.

3 | Standing side leg lift

Adding movement to the exercise makes balancing on one leg more difficult and also makes the exercise more "functional," since most balance challenges in real life come while you're in motion.

Starting position: Stand up straight, feet together and weight evenly distributed on both feet. Relax your arms at your sides.

Movement: Lift your right foot out to the side a few inches off the floor, shifting your weight over to your left leg. Lift your arms out to your sides to help you balance. Hold. Return to the starting position, then repeat with your left foot.

Reps: 1

Sets: 1–3

Hold: 5–30 seconds

Tips and techniques:

- Maintain good posture throughout by keeping your chest lifted, your shoulders down and back, and your abdominal muscles braced.
- Tighten the buttock of the standing leg to help you balance.
- Keep your toes and knees pointing forward.

Make it easier: Keep the toes of your raised leg lightly touching the floor.

Make it harder: Hold for 60 seconds; close your eyes.

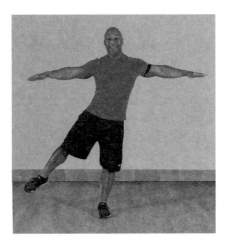

4 | Back leg lift

These leg lifts not only improve your balance, but also firm up your gluteal muscles.

Starting position: Stand up straight, feet together and weight evenly distributed on both feet. Relax your arms at your sides.

Movement: Lift your right foot straight behind you a few inches off the floor, shifting your weight over to your supporting leg. Lift your arms out to your sides to help you balance. Hold. Return to the starting position, then repeat with your left foot.

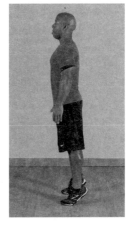

Reps: 1

Sets: 1–3

Hold: 5–30 seconds

Tips and techniques:

- Maintain good posture throughout by keeping your chest lifted, your shoulders down and back, and your abdominal muscles braced.
- Don't bend forward as you lift your leg.

Make it easier: Keep the toes of your raised leg lightly touching the floor.

Make it harder: Hold for 60 seconds; close your eyes.

5 | Heel raise with balance

This exercise, which you can do anywhere, builds strength in your calves while honing balance.

Starting position: Stand up straight, feet hip-width apart and weight evenly distributed on both feet. Put your arms at your sides.

Movement: Lift your heels until you're standing on the balls of your feet. Try to balance evenly without allowing your ankles to roll inward or outward. Hold. Lower your heels to the floor, maintaining good posture as you do.

Reps: 10

Sets: 1–3

Tempo: 2–2–2

Tips and techniques:

- In the starting position, think of each foot as forming a rectangle and stand with your weight evenly distributed on all four corners. When lifting, try to balance evenly on the front two corners.
- Tighten your abdominal and buttocks muscles as you balance on the balls of your feet.
- Imagine you have a string at the top of your head pulling you up to stand tall.

Make it easier: Don't lift your heels as high.

Make it harder: Hold for four to eight counts; close your eyes. ▼

Bonus: 3-Minute Cardio Interval Workout

This is the perfect workout when you're crunched for time or need a quick energy boost. Research shows that even short bursts of high-intensity exercise lead to improvements in cardio fitness. You can break up this workout into one-minute bursts three times a day (just do one exercise each time) and still get benefits. These "exercise snacks," as some researchers call such mini-workouts, have been found to help boost cardio fitness, improve blood sugar control, and enhance muscle function.

What makes these exercises high-intensity is that each one incorporates hops. However, you alternate the exercises with low-intensity marching in place, turning this into an interval workout.

Instructions: Warm up by doing 10 to 12 repetitions of each exercise at an easy pace without hopping. Then, do each exercise for 30 seconds, followed by 30 seconds of easy marching in place to recover before performing the next exercise. If 30 seconds is too much for you, you can do 15 seconds of each exercise and then repeat the entire series. If you want a longer workout, you can repeat the series as many times as you like. Cool down afterward with a few minutes of easy marching in place.

What you need: Nothing.

1 | Knee lift with hop and pull-down

This exercise is like a standing crunch, working your abdominal muscles while building power and cardio fitness.

Starting position: Stand with your feet together and both arms extended overhead.

Movement: Hop onto your left foot, raising your right knee and pulling both arms down. Lower your right foot and raise your arms. Immediately, hop onto your right foot, raising your left knee and pulling your arms down. Continue alternating legs for 30 seconds.

Then march in place for 30 seconds before going on to the next exercise.

Tips and techniques:
- Keep your chest lifted and your shoulders back.
- Don't lean forward or back as you raise your knee.
- Pull your arms down with power.

Make it easier: Do the move without the hop.

Make it harder: Hop higher, hop faster, or do both.

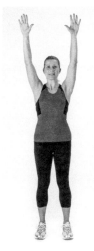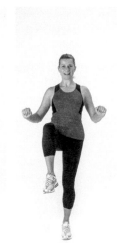

2 | Skater

This movement "wakes up" the lateral muscles that propel you side-to-side. Think of an Olympic speed skater to help you get into the spirit.

Starting position: Stand up straight with your feet hip-width apart and your arms at your sides.

Movement: Jump to the right as far as possible, landing on your right leg. Bring your left foot across behind you and swing your arms to the right as you bend your right knee into a lunge. Repeat, leaping to the left and lunging on your left leg with your right one behind you. Continue alternating directions for 30 seconds.

Then march in place for 30 seconds before going on to the next exercise.

Tips and techniques:
- Keep your chest and head lifted as you lunge.
- As you lunge, your knee should be aligned over your foot so you can see your toes if you look down.
- Tighten your abdominal muscles.

Make it easier: Step to the side instead of hopping. Make the lunge smaller. Or don't lunge at all; simply tap your foot behind you.

Make it harder: Make your hops bigger. Go faster. Lunge lower.

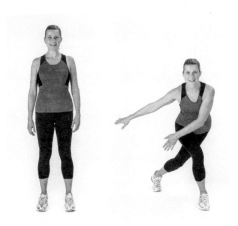

3 | Step-back lunge

This lunge puts the emphasis on controlling backward motion—something you probably don't do often—and helps develop key hip muscles for better stability.

Starting position: Stand up straight with your feet hip-width apart and your arms at your sides.

Movement: Step as far back as possible with your left foot and bend your right knee into a lunge. As you step back, swing your arms forward, elbows bent, to help you balance. Then, jump to bring your feet together. Repeat, stepping back with your right foot and then jumping to bring your feet together. Continue alternating legs for 30 seconds.

Then march in place for 30 seconds.

Tips and techniques:
- Keep your chest and head lifted as you lunge.
- As you lunge, your knee should be aligned over your foot so you can see your toes if you look down.
- Tighten your abdominal muscles.

Make it easier: Bring your feet together with a step instead of a jump. Make the lunge smaller. Or don't lunge at all; simply tap your foot behind you.

Make it harder: Move your foot back with a jump rather than a step, and then jump again to bring your feet together. ▼

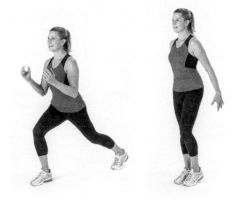

Special thanks to Michele Stanten, the fitness consultant for this report, for demonstrating most of the exercises and stretches depicted here. Master trainer Josie Gardiner demonstrated the Warm-up. Philip Penney is featured in the basic-level Strength Workout. The Balance Workout features trainer RaShaun Smith, and the first exercise in the challenge-level Core Workout shows Cynthia Roth.

Resources

Organizations

American Academy of Physical Medicine and Rehabilitation
9700 W. Bryn Mawr Ave., Suite 200
Rosemont, IL 60018
847-737-6000
www.aapmr.org

This national professional organization for physiatrists—medical doctors trained in physical medicine and rehabilitation—provides information on conditions such as low back pain, neck pain, and osteoarthritis. A referral service on the website can help you locate a physiatrist near you (go to the "About physiatry" pull-down menu, and click on "Find PM&R physician").

American College of Sports Medicine
401 W. Michigan St.
Indianapolis, IN 46202
317-637-9200
www.acsm.org

ACSM is a nonprofit association that educates and certifies fitness professionals, such as personal trainers, and offers information to the public on various types of exercise. A referral service on the website locates ACSM-certified personal trainers (go to the "Get & Stay Certified" pull-down menu, and click on "Find a Pro").

American Council on Exercise
4851 Paramount Drive
San Diego, CA 92123
888-825-3636 (toll-free)
www.acefitness.org

ACE is a nonprofit organization that promotes fitness and offers educational materials for consumers and professionals. The website includes a library of free exercise videos and a referral service to locate ACE-certified personal trainers and health coaches.

Institute of Lifestyle Medicine
Spaulding Rehabilitation Hospital Boston
300 First Ave.
Charlestown, MA 02129
617-952-6016
www.instituteoflifestylemedicine.org

The institute seeks to reduce the prevalence of lifestyle-related disease by changing behaviors. Physicians work with patients to change lifestyle choices that damage health and longevity. The website offers resources on stress management, nutrition, and physical activity.

National Institute on Aging
Building 31, Room 5C27
31 Center Drive, MSC 2292
Bethesda, MD 20892
800-222-2225 (toll-free)
www.nia.nih.gov/health/exercise-physical-activity

Part of the National Institutes of Health, the National Institute on Aging offers exercises, motivational tips, and free resources to help older adults get ready, start exercising, and keep going.

Special Health Reports

The following Special Health Reports from Harvard Medical School provide more ways to work out and get fit with body-weight exercises. To order, call 877-649-9457 (toll-free) or go to www.health.harvard.edu/special-health-reports.

A Beginner's Guide to Running: A gradual program to get you up to speed
(Harvard Medical School, 2020)

Better Balance: Simple exercises to improve stability and prevent falls
(Harvard Medical School, 2017)

Cardio Exercise: 7 workouts to boost energy, fight disease, and help you live longer
(Harvard Medical School, 2018)

Intermediate Yoga: Deepen your practice to find more strength, flexibility, energy, and happiness
(Harvard Medical School, 2021)

An Introduction to Tai Chi: A gentle exercise program for mental and physical well-being
(Harvard Medical School, 2017)

An Introduction to Yoga: Improve your strength, balance, flexibility, and well-being
(Harvard Medical School, 2020)

The Joint Pain Relief Workout: Healing exercises for your shoulders, hips, knees, and ankles
(Harvard Medical School, 2021)

Stretching: 35 stretches to improve flexibility and reduce pain
(Harvard Medical School, 2017)

Walking for Health: Why this simple activity could be your best health insurance
(Harvard Medical School, 2019)